DATE OF RETURN
UNLESS RECALLED BY LIBRARY

PLEASE TAKE GOOD CARE OF THIS BOOK

D1357549

LIVING THERAPY SERIES

Responding to a Serious Mental Health Problem

Person-centred dialogues

Richard Bryant-Jefferies

Radcliffe Publishing
Oxford • Seattle

Radcliffe Publishing Ltd
18 Marcham Road
Abingdon
Oxon OX14 1AA
United Kingdom

www.radcliffe-oxford.com
Electronic catalogue and worldwide online ordering facility.

© 2005 Richard Bryant-Jefferies

All rights reserved. No part of this publication may be reproduced, stored in a retrieval system or transmitted, in any form or by any means, electronic, mechanical, photo-copying, recording or otherwise, without the prior permission of the copyright owner.

British Library Cataloguing in Publication Data

A catalogue record for this book is available from the British Library.

ISBN 1 85775 703 3

59 73A

Typeset by Aarontype Ltd, Easton, Bristol
Printed and bound by TJ International Ltd, Padstow, Cornwall

Contents

Foreword

Having worked as a medical doctor (GP) in Ireland for 15 years, I realised that I needed to re-train in order to work effectively with people experiencing mental health problems. I therefore undertook and completed an MA in humanistic and integrative psychotherapy to address the deficits in my medical training. I believe that a person-centred approach to mental health is a pre-requisite to effective mental health work.

Within the mental health services, people experiencing serious and prolonged mental health problems are typically treated primarily – and often solely – with medication. The presumption is often made that therapy and psychosocial interventions for mental health experiences such as psychosis and paranoia could not possibly have anything to offer. Consequently, counsellors and psychotherapists do not tend to work regularly with people experiencing serious and enduring mental health problems.

Therapists tend to be less confident about working with people experiencing severe mental health problems. Many therapists do not gain sufficient experience in this work to understand such experiences and to become comfortable in this area of work. Within some counselling and psychotherapy training programmes, major mental health problems such as psychosis and paranoia are not considered in great detail, seen primarily as falling within the remit of psychiatry and medication only.

This is unfortunate. There is considerable scope for therapists to work with experiences such as hallucinations, delusions, paranoia, and with the experiences of people diagnosed as having bipolar disorder. Such experiences are typically viewed as meaningless, purposeless; as something to be eradicated as quickly as possible. I share the author's view that on the contrary, these experiences do indeed make sense and can be engaged with in therapy. These experiences reveal something important about that person and how they are in their world, albeit if sometimes presented in an indirect and metaphorical fashion.

Serious mental health problems tend to be seen primarily as medical problems. However, the person experiencing mental health problems has an existence, a life beyond their diagnosis. People become unwell within the contexts and systems in which they live. A mental healthcare system which does not sufficiently take these systems into account is inevitably limited in its capacity to help people recover.

In this book, Richard Bryant-Jefferies outlines in considerable detail the value of a person-centred approach to severe mental health problems. The detail is important; he pays great attention to the subtle nuances of relationship which are often missed within mental healthcare but which can be profoundly important to people's relationships, life and mental health.

The author takes the reader chronologically through the journey of mother and son. Included in this journey are aspects of the counsellor's own experience of the journey, including their supervision. As the story unfolds, the reader gets a real sense of the journey of both client and therapist. Richard Bryant-Jefferies provides insights into important aspects of relationships which therapists can work with productively within the relationship network of people experiencing severe mental health problems. What is also helpful and insightful is the fact that the mother is a Muslim woman with multicultural and religious issues being addressed within the therapeutic process.

This book will be of considerable interest to therapists and other health and social care professionals working within mental health who either regularly come into contact with people experiencing severe mental health problems, or who would be interested in increasing their understanding of this demanding but rewarding area. It will also be of interest to clients, to trainers and trainees as material for informing the training process.

Terry Lynch
Psychotherapist and GP
Limerick, Ireland
January 2005

Terry Lynch is the author of *Beyond Prozac: Healing Mental Distress* (2004) published by PCCS Books.

Foreword

Substance use and its impact on the mental health of young people is a growing problem. Young people today are subjected to, and are having to cope with, a range of difficulties and pressures. Many choose to use substances as a way of coping and of satisfying certain needs. These include a sense of belonging to peer groups, a way of dealing with difficult emotions, a way of experiencing highs and lows, something to do when feeling bored and needing excitement. Much of this is natural and normal adolescent experimental, adaptational and developmental behaviour; however, in the context of drug availability, and a culture of use amongst young people, serious negative consequences can arise. Sadly, the young people that I work with within Child and Adolescent Mental Health Services (CAMHS) very often present their substance use as having a very specific purpose, that of fulfilling a psychological need. They are often on the way to developing a firmly established habit.

In this book, Richard Bryant-Jefferies describes not only working with Ali, an older teenager who has a history of problematic cannabis use leading him to psychotic experiencing, but also of working with his mother who is in need of support as she tries to cope with the impact of his mental states on his behaviour within the family home. This, in my experience, is an all too common problem. The family system has to be taken into account in order to appreciate the factors contributing to the complexity of the problems that have arisen, and to identify what supportive systems are present to resolve the difficulties they face.

As a mother and a Muslim myself, I appreciate the fact that the author has set the narrative within a religious context. Here the mother has a Muslim faith and this informs her attitude and commitment to the family system and to her role as mother. We see the counsellor working with some of these issues, within the context of a society where there is much misunderstanding and misrepresentation of Islamic belief.

I have spent the last four years establishing a service for young people who are using drugs and who are referred to CAMHS with complex needs, including mental health issues. It has been a demanding and yet enormously fulfilling area of work. A worrying trend amongst young people is the high level of cannabis and/or alcohol use, and in particular the stronger varieties of cannabis now available and the culture of binge drinking until they are 'off their faces'. This substance use impacts on lifestyle, health and relationships and, in my experience, there is a sense for many young people of not having their difficulties and issues taken seriously, particularly within the family.

It leaves me feeling that young people need to understand themselves more, so that they can appreciate the harm that substance use is having on them. Often there has to be a realisation that mood changes, anxiety and depression are normal features of life, to be borne and managed rather than immediately suppressed by trying to change the experiences through substance use. Young people often need someone to talk things through with and to help them make sense; not only of their lives, but of symptoms they may be experiencing which have a mental health component. However, I find that for many young people there is a marked reluctance to want to acknowledge any link between their substance use and their mental state.

For me, *Responding to a Serious Mental Health Problem* is a valuable text. It offers genuine insight into the impact of substances on adolescent mental health, relationships within the family, and how the person-centred approach can be applied in this area of work. It is a book that will have value in CAMHS and all settings where professionals are required to work with young people and families.

Movena Lucas
CAMHS Liaison Clinical Nurse Specialist in Substance Misuse
January 2005

Preface

From the start of my own training in person-centred counselling the problematic potential of the mother–son relationship, and the under-emphasis on this within material written for counsellors, has struck me. I sought to begin to address this in my previous book in the Living Therapy series: *Relationship Counselling: sons and their mothers*. In that I dealt with the process of a man breaking free from being the 'son' in order to claim his independence as a male adult in his own right, and the difficulties that can arise within this process.

In this book, I planned to write a reverse situation, focusing on working with a mother whose son was evidencing problems of dependency. However, as the book evolved, it became a somewhat different narrative. In Part 1 of the book, I concentrate on one client, Fareeda, in her struggle to cope with her son, Ali, who at 19 has an undiagnosed mental health problem and has turned to cannabis to self-medicate. The second part of the book describes Ali's experience of entering into a therapeutic encounter after having reached a crisis point himself, and how he then addresses not only his cannabis use but also his now fragile mental state and the experiential factors that contributed to its development.

I set out to explore what happens when sons deliberately choose lifestyles that involve maintaining an identity as a dependent son, choosing a way of being that, for whatever reason, involves not taking responsibility and expecting to be baled out by a mother who is caught in their own dependency trap. In such instances we see a mother being dragged down by the constant demands of a son who, in a certain sense, is unable, or unwilling, to grow up. Cycles of co-dependency develop. Mother and son are sometimes caught in a dance which enables both to cling to identities that perhaps should have passed away long ago – the son not wishing to affirm his identity as independent adult; the mother unwilling to let go of certain aspects of her self-concept or identity as 'mother' and create the space and the opportunity to embrace a fresh phase in her own life.

However, I have found myself with a narrative which explores a situation in which it is not that the son is unwilling, but is unable to break free of dependency due to his own state of mental health and his use of cannabis to try and ease the acute discomfort he is experiencing within himself. The questions that arise are many, and include, 'how does the mother who knows she is needed by her son – and genuinely so – also look after herself and acknowledge her needs in order to stay healthy and free?'. And, 'how will the son address his difficulties when opportunity is offered for this to occur?'. Finally, there is the issue of the mental health problem and the substance use, and how the counsellor works with this from a person-centred perspective.

I have deliberately added a further layer of material in this volume by making Fareeda, the mother, a Muslim woman who draws strength and direction from her Islamic faith, and brings some of her own cultural differences into the therapeutic encounter with her counsellor, Carla. Issues arise both within Fareeda and Carla in response to this. Carla discusses issues and the counselling process with her supervisor, William, which opens up for her a greater self-understanding and much to ponder on further in her quest to understand the therapeutic encounter. For Fareeda the ongoing question is present, rooted in her Islamic faith, 'what is it that Allah requires of me in serving His will?', and in particular in the context of the strong emphasis on the primacy of family within Islamic culture.

Fareeda comes originally from Mauritius. She left her family to come over to England, and initially stayed with her sister. It was a few years later that she met Chris and fell in love with him. Her parents were not really approving, but they accepted her decision. They were aware that her sister had already followed a similar route by then and so it was less of a surprise to them when Fareeda informed them of her relationship with Chris and their intention to get married. She was pregnant with Ali quite soon after and then later decided to have a second child. They agreed that he would have an English name, Adam. However, the relationship had strains that emerged over time, and particularly in relation to Ali's behaviour and state of mind, with Fareeda feeling increasingly torn between needing to be there for Ali but painfully aware that it meant less time for Adam.

In Part 2, Ali, who has in many ways a more secular view of life than his mother whilst also carrying a certain sense of Muslim identity, encounters Charlotte, an experienced person-centred counsellor who is working in a drug service to enhance her professional practice. Ali is keyworked by another member of the team, Desmond, who is offering a cognitive-behavioural response to Ali's mental health difficulties. The person-centred counselling offers Ali space to explore in a relational and unstructured way his own traumatic experiences, their effect on his mental health and his developed structure of self, and to which he also brings what would generally be diagnosed as psychotic experiences and behaviours.

This book does not in any way set out to portray a 'typical' family in which cross-cultural differences exist, and Fareeda is not intended to represent a typical Muslim woman. I do not want to get caught in stereotypes. Fareeda is an independent woman seeking the best for her son, and wanting the best for her family. She has established a life for herself in England and draws from her Islamic faith in the way she seeks to live her life. She has, however, reached a point in her life where she knows she needs to talk.

Included in this volume is material to inform the training process of counsellors and many others who seek to work with people experiencing these relational dynamics. *Responding to a Serious Mental Health Problem: person-centred dialogues* is intended as much for experienced counsellors as it is for trainees. It provides real insight into what can occur during counselling sessions. I hope it will raise awareness of, and inform, not only person-centred practice within this relational context, but also contribute to other theoretical approaches within the world of counselling and psychotherapy. Reflections on the therapeutic process and points for discussion are included at the end of each chapter to stimulate further thought and debate.

Responding to a Serious Mental Health Problem: person-centred dialogues will also be of value to the many healthcare and social care professionals who, whilst they may specialise in other areas such as substance misuse, stress, family therapy and couple-counselling, will find that the issues dealt with in this volume have impact on the work they are doing. For all these professionals, the text contributes to demystifying what can occur in therapy, and at the same time provides useful ways of working that may be used by professionals other than counsellors. The book may also have value for people who have the kind of problems that Ali is facing, or those, like Fareeda, who are struggling to cope. Potential clients will gain an insight into the process as well, although, of course, this is always an expression of the unique relationship between a counsellor and their client.

I hope that in this book I am able to address a range of themes and leave you, the reader, with much to reflect on.

Richard Bryant-Jefferies
January 2005

About the author

Richard Bryant-Jefferies qualified as a person-centred counsellor/therapist in 1994 and remains passionate about the application and effectiveness of this approach. Between early 1995 and mid-2003 Richard worked at a community drug and alcohol service in Surrey, though more recently he has been appointed to manage NHS substance misuse services as part of the Central and North West London Mental Health NHS Trust, in the Royal Borough of Kensington and Chelsea in London. He has experience of offering counselling and supervision in NHS, GP and private settings, and has provided training through 'alcohol awareness and response' workshops. He is also available to offer workshops/talks/discussion related to the material he has written in the Living Therapy book series (Radcliffe Publishing). He can be contacted at richard@bryant-jefferies.fsnet.co.uk and via his website at www.bryant-jefferies.freeserve.co.uk

Richard had his first book on a counselling theme published in 2001, *Counselling the Person Beyond the Alcohol Problem* (Jessica Kingsley Publishers), providing theoretical yet practical insights into the application of the person-centred approach within the context of the 'cycle of change' model that has been widely adopted to describe the process of change in the field of addiction. Since then he has been writing for the ongoing Living Therapy book series, producing the titles of person-centred dialogues on *Problem Drinking*, *Time-Limited Therapy in Primary Care*, *Counselling a Survivor of Child Sexual Abuse*, *Counselling a Recovering Drug User*, *Counselling Young People*, *Counselling for Progressive Disability* and *Relationship Counselling: sons and their mothers*. The aim of the series is to bring the reader a direct experience of the counselling process, an exposure to the thoughts and feelings of both client and counsellor as they encounter each other on the therapeutic journey, and an insight into the value and importance of supervision. The author is currently working on titles to address the application of person-centred therapy to working with victims of warfare, people with obesity problems, counselling in the NHS workplace, problem gambling and eating disorders.

Richard is keen to bring the experience of the therapeutic process, from the standpoint and application of the person-centred approach, to a wider audience. He is convinced that the principles and attitudinal values of this approach and the emphasis it places on the therapeutic relationship are key to helping people create greater authenticity in themselves and in their lives, leading to a fuller and more satisfying human experience. By writing fictional accounts to try and bring the therapeutic process alive, to help readers engage with the characters within the narrative – client, counsellor and supervisor – he hopes to take the reader on a journey into the counselling room. Whether we think of it as pulling back the curtains or opening a door, it is about enabling people to access what can and does occur within the therapeutic process.

Acknowledgements

Working in the field of mental health is challenging, and additionally so when working with people whose lives are affected by substance use as well. I wish to thank the many people over the years who have contributed to my own experience and understanding of this area of work, fellow professionals and clients.

I would particularly like to thank and acknowledge the contribution of Movena Lucas to this book. Her experience as a mental health nurse, clinical nurse specialist in adult substance misuse and in offering specialist substance misuse liaison work with young people in a Child and Adolescent Mental Health Service, has been invaluable. Her additional insight as a Muslim woman and mother has also been extremely helpful in the writing of this book. I also wish to thank her for contributing a Foreword.

I also wish to express my appreciation to Terry Lynch for his Foreword, drawing as he has from his own experience as both psychotherapist and GP. His views strongly resonate with my own and I thank him for sharing them.

I wish to thank and acknowledge Sally Mulliner, a person-centred therapist who read through a draft of this book and contributed her own thoughts and experiences both as a therapist and as a mother who herself has a son who has mental health problems who has used substances. I am grateful to her son, Nick Springsguth, for his helpful comments on specific parts of the text. I would also like to thank Fatima Elguenuni for her valuable comments and insight on this volume from her perspective as an Islamic counsellor.

Finally, I am again indebted to Maggie Pettifer, and other members of the editorial and production team at Radcliffe Publishing. Their continued support for the Living Therapy series is obviously crucially important. Like me, they recognise that this narrative or dialogue style of presenting a therapeutic approach is an effective way of enabling readers to gain an understanding of a theoretical approach through engaging a process of counselling and supervision.

Introduction

The aim of the Living Therapy series is to offer the reader an opportunity to experience and to appreciate, through the use of dialogue, some of the diverse and challenging issues that can arise during counselling (Bryant-Jefferies, 2003a, 2003b, 2004). The success of the preceding volumes, and the appreciative comments received from readers and made by independent reviewers, is encouragement enough to seek to extend this style into other issues and areas of counselling. Again and again people remark on how readable and accessible these books are. This is particularly heartening. I want the style to draw people into the narrative and help them to feel engaged with the characters and the therapeutic process. I want it to be what I would term 'an experiential read'.

The complex relationship between mental illness and close family relationships, such as that between a mother and son, is a theme that I have certainly witnessed and been involved in as a counsellor. Issues of co-dependency, as both the mother and the son cling to roles that enable them to maintain certain facets of their natures and beliefs about themselves, can be potently present. An intergenerational psychological and behavioural dance is established and it becomes increasingly difficult to break free of the established relational rhythm. And yet there can come a point at which the mother will need to claim her independence and, by so doing, free the son to do the same. Or vice versa. Either way, someone has to change. It becomes painful and traumatic when the changes within each person do not coincide. This process, however, is further complicated where a mental health problem is involved.

With increasing numbers of young people using substances, and arguably more powerful substances, and from an earlier age, there has to be an expectation that more and more families are going to find themselves affected by a young person's substance use. How will the family respond? What role will each person take? Who will be supportive of the young person? Will this support, though, simply become more of a process of rescuing them from the effects of their damaging choices and in effect becoming a process of enabling the young person to continue with their use? And who will reject them, want to remove them from the family system completely, which can also end up enabling the substance misuse to continue and perhaps develop further?

In my experience as a therapist I have seen how parents can be split, with a mother often (though not always) struggling to support the son whose lifestyle has become increasingly problematic. They are pulled into a time-consuming role, perhaps we should say an all-consuming role, for if they cannot maintain boundaries and their own wellbeing then they will become consumed by the need of the young person and the demand within themselves to respond to that need. And yet, as in the story in this book, there will be times when the needs of the young person are justified. A young person with a mental health problem will need extra support and attention, and may well need a strong parent (or parents) to ensure that their needs are being met by mental health services. Nevertheless, patterns of relationship will evolve and may, in time, still become psychologically problematic, with a certain degree of dependence normalised within the young person's structure of self.

As with the other volumes of the Living Therapy series, this book is composed of fictitious dialogues between fictitious clients and their counsellors, and between the counsellors and their supervisors. Within the dialogues are woven the reflective thoughts and feelings of these different characters, along with boxed comments on the process and references to person-centred theory. By introducing the mother, Fareeda, as a Muslim woman, it affords an opportunity for her to bring a measure of her own rich cultural and religious beliefs into the therapeutic arena. Her son, Ali, is not simply using cannabis, he has a history of mood disorders, linked to a history of being bullied as a child, and of a lack of effective and consistent psychiatric care. His mental health deteriorates as he moves into using an arguably stronger form of cannabis – the exact science around this remains a topic of debate. Whilst there is some agreement that 'skunk' cannabis is more hallucinogenic than the 'pot', 'weed' or 'marijuana' that most people associate with cannabis, the degree remains debatable. However, some people do seem to find themselves more severely affected by 'skunk' cannabis. What is perhaps worth saying is that any shift towards using a more powerful drug, with more intense, adverse effects on the person, has to raise concerns, particularly when we are talking about young people who are still passing through their developmental stages of life. Physical and psychological development is occurring and drugs of this nature can only have an effect; the questions remain how much of an effect, and what might the long-term significance be for that young person's development?

Fareeda's counsellor, Carla, is forced to confront some of her own issues concerning race, religious and cultural differences, and treatment responses to mental health problems including the process of diagnosis. Carla's supervisor, William, offers her the space to explore these in supervision and supports her in clarifying her thoughts, feelings and reactions; freeing her to be more present, congruent and empathic towards her client.

For Ali's counsellor, Charlotte, there are issues associated with working with a client who evidences psychotic states within the counselling session which she takes to her supervisor, Matt. What are the boundaries to her competence? Can she maintain a therapeutic alliance with a client whose inner frame of reference is extended beyond anything that she feels able to relate to? What happens when a client's inner world extends beyond the horizon of that of the counsellor?

Clearly these are big issues to deal with and I do not seek to provide all the answers. Rather, I want to convey something of the process of working with the material that arises so that the reader may be stimulated into processing their own reactions and thereby gain insight into themselves and their practice. Often it will simply lead to more questions which I hope will prove stimulating to the reader and encourage them to think through their own position and boundary of competence.

The book has been written with the aim of demonstrating the counsellor's application of the person-centred approach (PCA) – a theoretical approach to counselling that has, at its heart, the power of the relational experience. It is this relational experience which I believe to be at the very heart of effective therapy, contributing to the possibility of releasing the client to realise greater potential for authentic living. The approach is widely used by counsellors working in the UK today: in a membership survey in 2001 by the British Association for Counselling and Psychotherapy, 35.6 per cent of those responding claimed to work to the person-centred approach, while 25.4 per cent identified themselves as psychodynamic practitioners. However, whatever the approach, it seems to me that the relationship is the key factor in contributing to a successful outcome – though this must remain a very subjective concept for who, other than the client, can really define what experience is to be taken as a measure of a successful outcome?

The reader may find it takes a while to adjust to the dialogue format. Many of the responses offered by the counsellors, Carla and Charlotte, are reflections of what their respective clients, Fareeda and Ali, have said. This is not to be read as conveying a simple repetition of the clients' words. Rather, the counsellors seek to voice empathic responses, often with a sense of 'checking out' that they are hearing accurately what the clients are saying. The client says something; the counsellor then conveys that they have heard it, sometimes with the same words, sometimes including a sense of what they feel is being communicated through the client's tone of voice, facial expression, or simply the atmosphere of the moment. The client is then enabled to confirm that he has been heard accurately, or to correct the counsellor in their perception. The client may then explore more deeply what they have been saying or move on, in either case with a sense that they have been heard and warmly accepted. To draw this to the reader's attention, I have included some of the inner thoughts and feelings that are present within the individuals who form the narrative.

Training and awareness-raising workshops are to be encouraged to enable the professional to develop a fuller understanding of issues concerning racial, ethnic, cultural and religious differences, as well as a deeper knowledge of the impact of substance misuse on the mental health of a young person, particularly where there have been indications of a developing mental health problem.

All characters in this book are fictitious and are not intended to bear resemblance to any particular person or persons.

Supervision

The supervision sessions are included to offer the reader insight into the nature of therapeutic supervision in the context of the counselling profession, a method of supervising that I term 'collaborative review'. For many trainee counsellors, the use of supervision can be something of a mystery, and it is hoped that this book will go a long way to unravelling this. In the supervision sessions I seek to demonstrate the application of the supervisory relationship. My intention is to show how supervision of the counsellor is very much a part of the process of enabling them to be professionally and personally effective in their work with clients.

Many professions do not recognise the need for some form of personal and process supervision, and often what is offered is only line management. However, counsellors are required to receive regular supervision in order to explore the dynamics of the relationship with the client, the impact of the work on the counsellor and on the client, to receive support, and to provide an opportunity for an experienced co-professional to monitor the supervisee's work in relation to ethical standards and codes of practice. The supervision sessions are included because they are an integral part of the therapeutic process. It is also hoped that they will help readers from other professions to recognise the value of some form of supportive and collaborative supervision in order to help them become more authentically present with their own clients.

I also favour an approach that is of a collaborative nature which I describe as a process of 'collaborative review'. Merry (2002, p. 173) describes what he terms 'collaborative inquiry' as a 'form of research or inquiry in which two people (the supervisor and the counsellor) collaborate or co-operate in an effort to understand what is going on within the counselling relationship and within the counsellor'. There are, of course, as many models of supervision as there are models of counselling. In this book the supervisor is seeking to apply the attitudinal qualities of the person-centred approach.

In the publication by Tudor and Worrall (2004) a number of theoretical and experiential strands are drawn together from within and outside of the person-centred tradition in order to develop a theoretical position on the person-centred approach to supervision. The book defines the necessary factors for effective supervision within this therapeutic discipline, and the respective responsibilities of both supervisor and supervisee in keeping with person-centred values and principles. They contrast person-centred working with other approaches to supervision and emphasise the importance of the therapeutic space as a place within which practitioners 'can dialogue freely between their personal philosophy and the philosophical assumptions which underlie their chosen theoretical orientation' (Tudor and Worrell, 2004, pp. 94–5). They affirm the values and attitudes of person-centred working (*see* page 5) and explore their application to the supervisory relationship.

It is the norm for all professionals working in the healthcare and social care environment in this age of regulation to be formally accredited or registered and to work to their own professional organisation's code of ethics or practice. For instance, registered counselling practitioners with the British Association for Counselling and Psychotherapy are required to have regular supervision and continuing professional development to maintain registration. Whilst professions other than counsellors will gain much from this book in their work with clients who present to them with the kinds of issues described herein, it is essential that they follow the standards, safeguards and ethical codes of their own professional organisation, and are appropriately trained and supervised to work with them on the issues that arise.

The person-centred approach

The person-centred approach (PCA) was formulated by Carl Rogers, and references are made to his ideas within the text of the book. However, it will be helpful for readers who are unfamiliar with this way of working to have an appreciation of its theoretical base.

Rogers proposed that certain conditions, when present within a therapeutic relationship, would enable the client to develop towards what he termed 'fuller functionality'. Over a number of years he refined these ideas, which he defined as 'the necessary and sufficient conditions for constructive personality change'. These he described as follows.

1   Two persons are in psychological contact.
2   The first, whom we shall term the client, is in a state of incongruence, being vulnerable or anxious.
3   The second person, whom we shall term the therapist, is congruent or integrated in the relationship.
4   The therapist experiences unconditional positive regard for the client.
5   The therapist experiences an empathic understanding of the client's internal frame of reference and endeavours to communicate this experience to the client.
6   The communication to the client of the therapist's empathic understanding and unconditional positive regard is to a minimal degree achieved. (Rogers, 1957, p. 96)

The first necessary and sufficient condition given for constructive personality change is that of 'two persons being in psychological contact'. However, although he later published this as simply 'contact' (Rogers, 1959), it is suggested (Wyatt and Sanders, 2002, p. 6) that this was actually written in 1953–4. They quote Rogers as defining contact in the following terms: 'Two persons are in psychological contact, or have the minimum essential relationship when each makes a perceived or subceived difference in the experiential field of the other' (Rogers, 1959, p. 207). A recent exploration of the nature of psychological contact from a person-centred perspective is given by Warner (2002).

Rogers defined empathy as meaning 'entering the private perceptual world of the other ... being sensitive, moment by moment, to the changing felt meanings which flow in this other person ... It means sensing meanings of which he or she is scarcely aware, but not trying to uncover totally unconscious feelings' (Rogers, 1980, p. 142). It is a very delicate process, and it provides, I believe, a foundation block. The counsellor's role is primarily to establish empathic rapport and communicate empathic understanding to the client.

Within this relationship the counsellor seeks to maintain an attitude of unconditional positive regard towards the client and all that they disclose. This is not 'agreeing with'; it is simply warm acceptance. Rogers writes, 'when the therapist is experiencing a positive, acceptant attitude towards whatever the client *is* at that moment, therapeutic movement or change is more likely to occur' (Rogers, 1980, p. 116). Mearns and Thorne suggest that 'unconditional positive regard is the label given to the fundamental attitude of the person-centred counsellor towards her client. The counsellor who holds this attitude deeply values the humanity of her client and is not deflected in that valuing by any particular client behaviours. The attitude manifests itself in the counsellor's consistent acceptance of and enduring warmth towards her client' (Mearns and Thorne, 1988, p. 59).

Last, but by no means least, is that state of being that Rogers referred to as congruence, but which has also been described in terms of 'realness', 'transparency', 'genuineness', 'authenticity'. Indeed Rogers wrote that '. . . genuineness, realness or congruence . . . this means that the therapist is openly being the feelings and attitudes that are flowing within at the moment . . . the term transparent catches the flavour of this condition' (Rogers, 1980, p. 115). Putting this into the therapeutic setting, we can say that 'congruence is the state of being of the counsellor when her outward responses to her client consistently match the inner feelings and sensations which she has in relation to her client' (Mearns and Thorne, 1999, p. 84). Interestingly, Rogers makes the following comment in his interview with Richard Evans that with regard to the three conditions, 'first, and most important, is therapist congruence or genuineness . . . one description of what it means to be congruent in a given moment is to be aware of what's going on in your experiencing at that moment, to be acceptant towards that experience, to be able to voice it if it's appropriate, and to express it in some behavioural way' (Evans, 1975).

I would suggest that any congruent expression by the counsellor of their feelings or reactions has to emerge through the process of being in therapeutic relationship with the client. It is a disciplined response and not an open door to endless self-disclosure. Congruent expression is perhaps most appropriate and therapeutically valuable where it is informed by the existence of an empathic understanding of the client's inner world, and is offered in a climate of a genuine warm acceptance towards the client. The person-centred approach regards the relationship that we have with our clients, and the attitude that we hold within that relationship, to be key factors. In my experience, many adult psychological difficulties develop out of life experiences that involve problematic, conditional or abusive relational experiences. This can be centred in childhood or later in life. What is significant is that the individual is left, through relationships that have a negative conditioning effect, with a distorted perception of themselves and their potential as a person. I have seen many people who have learned from childhood experience beliefs such as 'my role is to care for others, whatever the cost to me', 'no one seemed to be there for me when I was a child but I will never be like that towards my children', or 'no one was there for me, I never felt loved; I guess I'm unlovable'.

The result is a conditioned sense of self, with the individual then thinking, feeling and acting in ways that enable them to maintain these self-beliefs and meanings within their learned concept of self. This conditioned sense of self is then lived out, possibly throughout life, the person seeking to satisfy what they have come to believe about themselves: needing, for instance, to care either because it has been normalised, or in order to prove to themselves and the world that they are a 'good' person. They will need to maintain this conditioned sense of self and the sense of satisfaction that this gives them when it is lived out because they have developed such a strong identity with it.

There is also, inevitably, the 'nature' or 'nurture' debate to address. However, there is much already written on this topic and it is not an aspect I will be dwelling on. Why, though, does the debate always seem to be polarised in 'either, or'? Why not 'both', thereby adding to the complexity and diversity of what it is to be a human being, having natural and unique potential which then becomes encouraged, thwarted or distorted by the nature of the nurturing that is available; or the experience of problems within the brain chemistry and functioning, which simply make some experiences and behaviours so difficult to manage, and also difficult to understand and empathise with.

Obviously, relationships between parents and their offspring will be a major conditioning factor in the development of the child on the journey towards adulthood. However, relationships with peers – with whom a child or young person will spend much of their time, for instance, at school – will also be extremely significant. We only have to think about the effects of bullying and abuse that can take place to know that people can be left severely and adversely affected in their psychological development. We learn about ourselves through the reactions of those closest to us. Their consistent presence means that our view of ourselves is shaped by the experiences we have and the meanings that we attribute to them. The child's first relationship is with his or her mother. Whilst her response is contributing to the child's emerging structure of self, it is likely to have been shaped itself through her own experience of being related to as a child and how that experience was internalised and what meanings were attributed to this.

Clearly a rejecting response, or where a parent may necessarily need to be occupied with another member of the family (perhaps a newborn brother or sister), or other matters (lack of physical or emotional availability due to work, perhaps, or other activities and pressures), can have a significant impact and will set up a chain reaction of 'self-beliefs' in the child that will be very different from those that develop where time is available for the child to receive empathy, love, warmth, honesty and trust. Without these, the child can be left with a damaged sense of self which will then find expression in a range of attitudes and behaviours that are perhaps more likely to be problematic and difficult. Or, what of the child for whom the brightly coloured toys or the vivid images of television and videos are the main source of stimulation and relationship, with reduced levels of actual heartfelt human contact? Whilst it might stimulate visual and aural receptors in the brain, it seems likely that other areas may, through deficiency of stimulation, be impaired in their development. If a child does not experience love, or this is not constantly reinforced, do they then develop an impaired ability to experience love and, as a result, find it more difficult to express love to others?

Then there is the wider circle of family members, and family friends, and then the social reaction of others, of people previously not known. Any developed feelings of being accepted, valued and of worth may be significantly undermined by the reactions of a child or young person's social world. Where a child is exposed to difficult relational experiences in, for instance, school settings, in the form of bullying and racial harassment, and if for whatever reason the child feels unable to take the effects of this experience to anyone who can respond in an appropriate and heartfelt manner, and who can act to put a stop to it, then the negative internalising and symbolising process is deepened, with the effects taking deeper root in the child's developing structure of self. The impact of this can be lasting and, as presented in this volume, generate effects which can arguably be the basis for experiences and behaviours that are likely to be associated with a mental health diagnosis. They may lose self-esteem to the point that in adulthood much work is required in order to recover it. For others, they may internalise the realisation that the only way to survive is to become the bully themselves, their frustrations in childhood getting lived out through adult relationships, for instance, domestically, socially or in the workplace.

Having established a structure of self and a way of being that is rooted in a negative set of childhood, relational experiences, it may then take a therapeutic encounter later in life to unravel the damage and help them to free themselves from views that they have about themselves and relationships, and the associated behaviours that have developed.

Mental health and diagnosis

Rogers wrote of the process of psychological breakdown and disorganisation. He expressed four stages to this process, the first two stages of which 'may be illustrated by anxiety-producing experiences in therapy, or by acute psychotic breakdowns'.

1 If the individual has a large or significant degree of *incongruence between self and experience* and if a significant experience demonstrating this *incongruence* occurs suddenly, or with a high degree of obviousness, then the organism's process of *defense* is unable to operate successfully.
2 As a result *anxiety is experienced*, as the *incongruence* is subceived. The degree of anxiety is dependent upon the extent of the *self-structure* which is *threatened*. (Rogers, 1959, pp. 228–9)

As a result of this process, Rogers then went on to describe the effects this has on the individual's self-structure and subsequent behaviour. He writes the following.

3 The process of defense being unsuccessful, the *experience* is *accurately symbolised* in *awareness*, and the gestalt of the *self-structure* is broken by this *experience* of the *incongruence* in *awareness*. A state of disorganisation results.
4 In such a state of disorganisation the organism behaves at times in ways which are openly consistent with experiences which have hitherto been distorted or denied to awareness. At other times the self may temporarily regain regnancy, and the organism may behave in ways consistent with it. Thus in such a state of disorganisation, the tension between the concept of self (with its included distorted perceptions) and the experiences which are not accurately symbolised or included in the concept of self, is expressed in a confused regnancy, first one and then the other supplying the 'feedback' by which the organism regulates behaviour. (Rogers, 1959, p. 229)

It then becomes an interesting question to consider what impact a mood-altering substance might have on this process and which substances (illicit or prescribed) will have the tendency to open up an individual's awareness to the incongruence within their self-structure, and which will in some way enhance the internal defences. Could it be that for some people, the use of cannabis, particularly skunk cannabis, weakens the defences and causes incongruence to break into awareness, thereby precipitating a psychotic event? This would suggest that such events are more likely for those whose structure of self is riddled with incongruence rooted in early life experience.

Interestingly, Rogers then cites sodium pentathol therapy, under the influence of which the client could reveal experiences that he had previously denied to himself, but which were clearly linked to 'incomprehensible elements in his behavior'. Faced with this material in his normal state of mind, the individual could no longer deny the authenticity of what had come into awareness and his 'defensive processes could not deny or distort the experience, and hence the self-structure was broken, and a psychotic break occurred' (Rogers, 1959, p. 229). Given the amount of drug use in society today, and the numbers of young people presenting with forms of mental disturbance, there is scope here for serious research. Certainly the fact that some people use cannabis without seemingly experiencing a problematic mental health reaction, whilst others do experience psychotic effects – and similarly with other substances – demands further investigation.

Let us move on, at this point, to a consideration of the person-centred view of the diagnostic process, particularly as it applies to the condition of a person's mental health. I have referred elsewhere (Bryant-Jefferies, 2003c) to the debate as to whether diagnosis can necessarily be trusted and empirical when it comes to mental health factors, drawing attention to Bozarth (2002), who refers to his own studies of particular diagnostic concepts which do not evidence the clustering of symptoms in a meaningful way (Bozarth 1998), and to those of others in relation to schizophrenia (Bentall, 1990; Slade and Cooper, 1979); depression (Hallett, 1990; Wiener, 1989); agoraphobia (Hallam, 1983), borderline personality disorder (Kutchins and Kirk, 1997); and panic disorder (Hallam, 1989).

Rogers also questioned the value of psychological diagnosis. He argued that it could place the client's locus of value firmly outside of themselves and definitely within the diagnosing 'expert', leaving the client at risk of developing tendencies of dependence and expectation that the 'expert' will have the responsibility of improving the client's situation (Rogers, 1951, p. 223). He also formulated the following propositional statements.

- Behaviour is caused, and the psychological cause of behaviour is a certain perception or a way of perceiving.
- The client is the only one who has the potentiality of knowing fully the dynamics of his perceptions and his behaviour.
- In order for behaviour to change, a change in perception must be *experienced*. Intellectual knowledge cannot substitute for this.
- The constructive forces which bring about altered perception, reorganisation of self, and relearning, reside primarily in the client, and probably cannot come from outside.
- Therapy is basically the experiencing of the inadequacies in old ways of perceiving, the experiencing of new and more accurate and adequate perceptions, and the recognition of significant relationship between perceptions.
- In a very meaningful and accurate sense, therapy *is* diagnosis, and this diagnosis is a process which goes on in the experience of the client, rather than in the intellect of the clinician. (Rogers, 1951, pp. 221–3)

Steve Vincent has drawn together some valuable passages from Rogers in relation to the question of diagnosis, emphasising that '*therapist* diagnosis, evaluation and prognosis clearly do not respect the inner resources of *clients* and their potential and capacity for self-direction, as there is an obvious implication that actually the therapist, not the client, knows best' (Vincent, 2005). He then quotes a passage from Rogers from his earlier days, yet a statement that stands the test of time, sounding with great clarity an essential person-centred perspective on this issue.

> If we can provide understanding of the way the client seems to himself at this moment, he can do the rest. The therapist must lay aside his pre-occupation with diagnosis and his diagnostic shrewdness, must discard his tendency to make professional evaluations, must cease his endeavours to formulate an accurate prognosis, must give up the temptation subtly to guide the individual, and must concentrate on one purpose only; that of providing deep understanding and acceptance of his attitudes consciously held at this moment by the client as he explores step by step into the dangerous areas which he has been denying to consciousness. (Rogers, 1946)

Lisbeth Sommerbeck, draws from her experience of working as a person-centred psychotherapist and supervisor in a psychiatric hospital in Denmark. She makes it very clear that 'psychiatric diagnosis is of no issue in client-centred theory and therapy'. She continues by stressing that 'the conditions necessary and sufficient for facilitation of the client's most constructive potentials are trusted to be the same for everybody, irrespective of diagnosis'. However, she also makes the important point that the client-centred therapist working in a psychiatric setting should not be ignorant about the diagnoses that are employed by others within that particular healthcare setting, or regard such diagnoses as unnecessary. 'In the medical model setting of a psychiatric hospital, for example, it is necessary for the client-centred therapist to acknowledge the necessity of psychiatric diagnostics for other professionals and to know about the main psychiatric diagnoses' (Sommerbeck, 2003, p. 33).

Rogers, in a letter quoted by Stevens (Rogers and Stevens, 1973, pp. 171–2), writes as follows.

> What does the word schizophrenic mean to me? To the extent that it has any definite meaning at all, it means that here is a person who is highly sensitive to his own inner experience and also to interpersonal relationships with others, who has been so defeated and traumatized in endeavouring to make use of his sensitivities that he has retreated both from his own experiencing and from any real contact with others. In addition, the word schizophrenic also means to me that anyone whose behaviour is deviant and who cannot be easily understood is tossed in this all encompassing basket.

On the same page, Stevens quotes from a letter by Gendlin, where he contributes a particularly important view, bringing the human and the relational elements alive to our interpretation of the way of being that may be diagnosed as schizophrenic.

> I believe that schizophrenia is *the absence of* (or greater narrowing of) that felt experiential interaction process which we are as people and which we feel as our concrete selves. When an individual is stuck in a hurtful relationship situation so that he can neither leave it nor feel and relate himself sufficiently to it, then he becomes deadened and empty inside, reports that he is 'not himself'. The ongoing feeling process on which we all rely inside becomes muddy, swampy, unreliable, or stopped, and feeling contents become stuck, frozen, unowned, seemingly alien, static places, rather than fluidly functioning feeling ... (Rogers and Stevens, 1973, pp. 171–2)

This definition of schizophrenia as an absence of a certain type of felt interaction (an absence rather than an illness or a content) has important consequences. It seems that we think of ourselves not so much as working with something ill in the person, but rather as providing the necessary personal relationship in the context of which someone can again come alive as a person.

This is a challenging and yet optimistic perspective, and fully in line with the person-centred view of the person as a process of being tending towards fullness, wholeness and complexity, a tendency that can tend towards fullest functionality within the experience of the relational experience that contains the core conditions of empathy, congruence and unconditional positive regard. The healing process that occurs through the constructive relational experience enables the 'damaged' individual to self-heal, to fill the gaps, the emptiness and the loneliness that can lie at the heart of some forms of mental disturbance. It is then not so much a case of there being a specific 'illness' to treat, but rather the need for a relational experience to encourage greater wholeness.

Nevertheless, there remains a belief that specific conditions respond to specific therapeutic treatments. Yet it has also been argued strongly that within the mental health context such specific treatments for specific dysfunctions are a myth (Bozarth, 2002). In his conclusion, Bozarth goes so far as to call for a 'radical restructuring of the mental health system (US) to accentuate the variables related to success. These are the common factor variables of therapist/ client relationship and emphasis on client resources and the client's frame of reference'. Elsewhere, Curtis Jenkins (2002) comments, with reference to Asay and Lambert (1999), that 'the reality is that most psychotherapy researchers now reluctantly agree that therapists themselves are more likely to be the cause of outcome variance than the style of therapy offered'. So rather than fit a particular treatment to a particular diagnosis – the traditional approach – we are best to consider matching a particular client to a particular therapist, a genuine person-to-person arrangement, for, in the final analysis, it is the relationship between two people that is arguably the most crucial and significant factor in successful outcome. And in making this decision it is crucial that the client is recognised as the person most able to judge as to the particular person that they wish to engage with in the therapeutic process. Interestingly, Mearns and Thorne express the opinion that 'congruence as a therapeutic condition becomes more critical with psychotic clients', a view that they emphasise being supported by the study of person-centred therapy with schizophrenic clients. They draw from Rogers (Rogers *et al.*, 1967, p. 86) in pointing out that 'those patients who perceived a high degree of congruence in their therapist were independently rated as showing the greatest degree of change. Furthermore, those patients who were in relationships where the therapist exhibited low congruence showed no change or even *regressive* change' (Mearns and Thorne, 1999, p. 105).

Personally, it seems that the therapeutic condition that is most effective for a given client will be that which is the opposite to what the client has been damaged by a lack of. So, the psychotic client who has developed high levels of incongruence will be most positively affected by the congruent therapist; the client who was adversely affected by a lack of warmth and prizing will require a therapist able to offer high levels of unconditional positive regard; the client who was not listened to or heard during their early development will need high levels of accurate, empathic understanding within their therapeutic experience; and the client who withdraws into their own reality and away from external contact will need a therapist who can work effectively within a relational experience of minimal psychological contact by staying close to the client without threatening to invade their psychological world. Is this too simplistic? I don't think so.

When working with clients who are evidencing 'psychotic' symptoms – withdrawal into a reality that seems alien to the socially accepted 'norm' – or who have a 'personality disorder' (where the personality characteristics, we might say the structure of self, have developed in such a way due to, for instance, often traumatic and undermining experiences, that the person's ability to function without constant distress or as a social being is greatly impaired), the counsellor can be greatly challenged. It can be, and often is, an intensely demanding, frustrating and disorientating experience. With regard to working with the psychotic client, Lambers writes of the challenge to the 'counsellor's ability to create the therapeutic conditions' and of the 'fundamental challenge to the therapist's understanding and expression of the conditions' (Lambers, 1994, p. 114). She writes of how, 'at the core of the self-concept of the client with personality disorder', there is 'a profound sense of worthlessness. A central issue in the counselling relationship is acceptance. The counsellor is likely to experience challenge of her ability to offer acceptance; the client will be challenged in his ability to experience being accepted' (Lambers, 1994, p. 120).

Lambers also draws attention to the importance of the therapeutic context with regard to this client group. She highlights Mearns' (1990) concept of a fourth condition (in addition to the three core conditions) of 'sufficiency of the therapeutic context' (Lambers, 1994, p. 115). By this is meant the need for consideration as to whether the usual 'therapeutic hour' is the most appropriate for the client, that there may be a need for more contact, perhaps more informal contact, and in an environment that has a greater 'holding effect' on the client – meeting a range of their basic needs. This might be represented by, for instance, a supported housing environment or residential, therapeutic community. It may well require other people working with the client, for instance a keyworker maintaining a holding role in relation to social and practical needs, leaving the counsellor free to concentrate on therapeutic work (though, of course, there is likely to be some degree of therapeutic overlap). My experience is of the need for greater flexibility – but this does not mean the counsellor is unboundaried. Perhaps shorter sessions will be more acceptable, or flexibility in the length of contact, negotiated within the process each time the client and counsellor meet.

I would like to end with a lengthy passage from Rogers and Stevens (1973, p. 154), taken from an abridged version of John Schlien's paper, 'A client-centered approach to schizophrenia: first approximation'*, as it seems to me to capture something extremely valuable when thinking about 'psychosis' and 'paranoia'.

> That which we call 'psychosis' is not a disease. It is a learned behaviour, exaggerated to a point of no return, i.e. where control is lost and the exaggerated behaviour 'takes on a life of its own' temporarily. Because this exaggeration is so overwhelming, so much beyond our ordinary capacity to assimilate, it appears to us that we are no longer dealing with, for instance, ordinary suspicion, but something *quite* different – 'paranoia'. Then it appears that psychosis is not of the same order, not on the same continuum, as 'normal' or 'neurotic' behaviour. But as psychotic behaviour becomes more common it is seen as a form of maladjustment similar in kind to lesser degrees of maladjustment, though so much greater in quantity that it seems different in *quality* too.

---

* This passage is taken from the abridged version which appears in: Rogers R and Stevens B (1973) *Person to Person: the problem of being human.* Souvenir Press, London. The full paper having appeared in: Burton A (ed.) (1961) *Psychotherapy of the Psychoses.* Basic Books.

He then continues to describe metaphorically how 'in one sense . . . it *is* different'.

> A boulder balanced on the edge of a precipice can be pressed ounce by measured ounce towards rolling off. Each ounce is just like the last, but when the quantity of pressure totals to the 'breaking point', the quality of the *consequences* changes radically. No longer will the relief or counterpressure of one ounce recover the balance. Even if the boulder is not smashed in the fall, an enormous effort is required to restore it to its original position. It is because of this effort (which so few can make, and so many need) that it is necessary to prevent the 'psychotic situation' in life. The 'psychotic situation' is a precondition to the psychotic state, which may or may not follow.

Further thoughts

Prior to the previous section addressing diagnosis, I mentioned the word 'love'. It is an important word, though not necessarily one used to describe therapeutic relationship. Patterson, however, gives a valuable definition of love as it applies to the person-centred therapeutic process. He writes, 'we define love as an attitude that is expressed through empathic understanding, respect and compassion, acceptance, and therapeutic genuineness, or honesty and openness towards others' (Patterson, 2000, p. 315). We all need love, but most of all we need it during our developmental period of life. The same author affirms that 'whilst love is important throughout life for the wellbeing of the individual, it is particularly important, indeed absolutely necessary, for the survival of the infant and for providing the basis for the normal psychological development of the individual' (Patterson, 2000, pp. 314–15).

It is my belief that by offering someone a non-judgemental, warm and accepting, and authentic relationship – in truth an experience of love (perhaps we need to speak more of therapeutic love) – then that person can grow into a fresh sense of self in which their potential as a person can become more fulfilled. Such an experience fosters an opportunity for the client to redefine themselves as they experience the presence of the therapist's congruence, empathy and unconditional positive regard. This process can take time. Often the personality change that is required to sustain a shift away from what have been termed 'conditions of worth' requires a lengthy period of therapeutic work, bearing in mind that the person may be struggling to unravel a sense of self that has been developed, sustained and reinforced for many decades of life.

The term 'conditions of worth' applies to the conditioning that is frequently present in childhood, and at other times in life, when a person experiences that their worth is conditional on their doing something, or behaving, in a certain way. This is usually to satisfy someone else's needs, and can be contrary to the client's own sense of what would be a satisfying experience. The values of others become a feature of the individual's structure of self. The person moves away from being true to themselves, learning instead to remain 'true' to their conditioned sense of worth. This state of being in the client is challenged by the person-centred therapist by offering them unconditional positive regard and warm acceptance. Such a therapist, by genuinely offering these therapeutic attitudes, provides the client with an opportunity to be exposed to what may be a new experience or one that in the past they have dismissed, preferring to stay with that which matches and therefore reinforces their conditioned sense of worth and sense of self. Unconditional positive regard and warm acceptance offered consistently over time can, and does, enable clients to begin to question their beliefs about themselves and to begin to build into their structure of self the capacity to see and experience themselves as being of value for who they are. It enables them to liberate themselves from the constraints of patterns of conditioning.

A crucial feature or factor in this process is the presence of what Rogers (1986) termed 'the actualising tendency', a tendency towards fuller and more complete personhood with an associated greater fulfilment of their potentialities. The role of the person-centred counsellor is to provide the facilitative climate within which this tendency can work constructively. The 'therapist trusts the actualizing tendency of the client and truly believes that the client who experiences the freedom of a fostering psychological climate will resolve his or her own problems' (Bozarth, 1998, p. 4). This is fundamental to the application of the person-centred approach. Rogers (1986, p. 198) wrote: 'the person-centred approach is built on a basic trust in the person ... (It) depends on the actualizing tendency present in every living organism – the tendency to grow, to develop, to realize its full potential. This way of being trusts the constructive directional flow of the human being towards a more complex and complete development. It is this directional flow that we aim to release.'

From this theoretical perspective we can argue that the person-centred counsellor's role is essentially facilitative. Returning to a topic previously referred to, the presence of a diagnosis becomes secondary to the simple fact that the client is attending with some degree of psychological discomfort that is manifesting through a set of symptoms and behaviours that have been diagnostically labelled as a specific 'illness'. Creating the therapeutic climate of empathic understanding, unconditional positive regard and authenticity creates a relational climate in which the client's own inherent capacity towards actualising their fuller potential as a person can become directed towards establishing a fresh sense of self that is liberated from the 'conditions of worth', perhaps rooted in traumatising experiences that are all too often at the root of psychological discomfort.

Whilst it is recognised that there will be certain conditions of mind which will require chemical interventions because the condition is the result of chemical imbalance or organic deficiencies, we should not allow this to blind us to the possibility that there are underlying environmental and experiential factors that have made a major contribution to a person's state of mind and emotion. I describe it thus because whilst the emphasis is on 'mental health', it is important to keep visible the fact that for many people their difficulties and psychological discomforts are strongly linked to difficult emotional experiencing. It is important to acknowledge that symptomology might be better seen as a kind of experiential flashing neon sign, drawing attention to the fact that something is wrong. If our treatment responses are simply concerned with turning off the flashing light because it is a problem to us, rather than seeking the underlying reason why it is flashing, then we have a system that goes no further than symptom management. Whilst this may well have a part to play in bringing a client symptom relief, it should not be confused with treatment of the underlying cause.

In addressing these factors the therapeutic relationship is central. A therapeutic approach such as person-centred affirms that it is not what you do so much as 'how you are' with your client that is therapeutically significant, and this 'how you are' has to be received by the client. Gaylin (2001, p. 103) highlights the importance of client perception. 'If clients believe that their therapist is working on their behalf – if they perceive caring and understanding – then therapy is likely to be successful. It is the condition of attachment and the perception of connection that have the power to release the faltered actualization of the self.' He goes on to stress how 'we all need to feel connected, prized – loved', describing human beings as 'a species born into mutual interdependence', and that there 'can be no self outside the context of others. Loneliness is dehumanizing and isolation anathema to the human condition. The relationship,' he suggests 'is what psychotherapy is all about.'

In a previous volume in this series I used the analogy of treating a wilting plant (Bryant-Jefferies, 2003c, p. 12). We can spray it with some specific herbicide or pesticide to eradicate a perceived disease that may be present in the plant, and that may be enough. But perhaps the true cause of the disease is that the plant is located in harsh surroundings, perhaps too much sun and not enough water, poor soil, near other plants that it finds difficulty in surviving so close to. Maybe by offering the plant a healthier environment that will facilitate greater nourishment according to the needs of the plant, it may reach its potential to become a strong, healthy plant. Yes, the chemical intervention may also be helpful, but if the true causes of the diseases are environmental – essentially the plant's relationship with that which surrounds it – then it won't actually achieve sustainable growth. We may not be able to transplant it, but we can provide water, nutrients and maybe shade from a fierce sun. Therapy, it seems to me, exists to provide this healthy environment within which the wilting client can begin the process of receiving the nourishment (in the form of healthy relational experience) that can enable them, in time, to become a more fully functioning person.

This is obviously a very brief introduction to the approach. Person-centred theory continues to develop as practitioners and theoreticians consider its application in various fields of therapeutic work and extend our theoretical understanding of developmental and therapeutic processes. At times it feels like it has become more than just individuals, rather it feels like a group of colleagues, based around the world, working together to penetrate deeper towards a more complete theory of the human condition. Person-centred or client-centred theory and practice has a key role in this process. It is an exciting time.

There is currently growing interest in, and much debate about, theoretical developments within the person-centred world and its application. Discussions on the theme of Rogers' therapeutic conditions presented by various key members of the person-centred community have been published (Bozarth and Wilkins, 2001; Haugh and Merry, 2001; Wyatt, 2001; Wyatt and Sanders, 2002).

Mearns and Thorne have produced a timely publication revising and developing key aspects of person-centred theory (2000). Wilkins has produced a book that addresses most effectively many of the criticisms levelled against person-centred working (2003). It seems to me that the relational component of the person-centred approach, based on the presence of the core conditions, is emerging strongly as a counter to the sense of isolation that frequently accompanies deep psychological and emotional problems, and which is a feature of materialistic societies as we enter the 21st century.

PART I

A mother seeks counselling

First contact

Fareeda was struggling. She knew things were getting out of hand but she could not see any way of being different. It seemed that so much of her life had been a succession of demands, and in many ways she was OK with that, it was the struggle that she felt she had with the healthcare system that got her down. At times it left her feeling so alone and doubting of what she believed, of what she knew to be true. Her faith had sustained her. Prayer had been an important part of her life as she sought reassurance and support from Allah (Arabic for God) in what she felt was right for her to do for the best for her eldest son, Ali.

She had realised some years ago that something was not quite right with her son. At first it had seemed that she was the only one to notice that he was always just that little bit louder, more intense, than his friends. She had noticed, too, how difficult at times he seemed to find it to settle down, and yet at other times he would seem so withdrawn. She could remember the first time that she had said to her sister that it seemed like he was two different people. At the time she did not really think much more about it, rather it was simply a passing comment. And yet . . .

As she looked back now she was so aware that in fact she had recognised something that was so much closer to the truth than she could then have imagined. The past four years had been a period of progressive difficulty; she often referred to it as like walking a tightrope, and yet not feeling able to step off it. It was as if she no longer had control over life, it was governed by whatever mood her elder son happened to be in at the time.

Fareeda was sitting at home looking at a card that a friend had given her. It didn't say a great deal, other than the name of a counsellor and the contact details, and the fact that she offered something called person-centred counselling. Fareeda didn't know what that was but the friend who had given her the card was quite insistent that she was good and came recommended.

The truth was that Fareeda was desperate. She wanted to talk to someone. She did not get much support at home. Her husband, Chris, Ali's father, tended to be distant. He didn't seem to have the same sense of family that she did. This had been, and still was, a disappointment to her, and something that she knew she found difficult. Chris also found it hard to accept and cope with Ali's difficulties.

They didn't often discuss the situation, not in a meaningful way. Any discussion tended to descend quickly into argument, with Chris taking the view that he should be kicked out. He didn't believe that Ali had a mental health problem, but rather that he was idle and needed to get himself a proper job and get his act together. Ali was now 19, soon to be 20, and Fareeda wondered and worried about what his future would hold for him.

It hadn't helped that there had never been a clear diagnosis so treatment was witheld. Right the way through, the professionals had thought that Ali was simply being a teenager, maybe extreme, but nevertheless, that he would change once he got older. Fareeda had fought this view, convinced that there was something more deep-seated. At weaker moments she had wondered whether she should accept the notion that he was simply being a difficult teenager, and that maybe it was the will of Allah for it to be the way that it was, being his way of testing her. But she couldn't feel comfortable with that. She knew instinctively something was not right, and the mood swings and the erratic behaviour remained. She knew she had to keep trying to help him.

Fareeda often spoke to her sister but she was always rather too good at giving advice. Fareeda felt she wanted someone to listen to her, not keep telling her what to do, which was often to accept things. She didn't accept things and she didn't want to be told what to do. She knew what she had to do. She was Ali's mother and she had to be there for him, wanted to be there for him. Now, she just wanted someone to talk to about how she was feeling. She wanted to unload. Her friend had told her that was what she had needed when she had been to see this counsellor whose name was printed on the card that she was now sitting and holding in front of her. Her friend had been quite persuasive as to how helpful it had been to just go and unload it all on a counsellor, a stranger, someone who wasn't going to keep giving you opinions and advice. Fareeda had thought about it. She trusted her friend, but she also was unsure as to whether she should be seeking out a Muslim counsellor. That did have an appeal, and yet she knew how much this counsellor had helped her friend – who was not a Muslim – and having someone recommended like that did somehow feel easier. She knew she had to make a decision, and the card was in her hand, and she knew she had to talk.

Fareeda reached for the phone and dialled the number on the card. The phone rang four times, there was a click and then a voice. 'Hello. This is Carla. Please don't hang up. I am sorry I cannot get to the phone just at the moment, but if you would like to leave your name and number I will call you back as soon as I can. If you are calling about the counselling service, please be assured that this answer machine will only be checked by me and therefore your message will be confidential. Thank you for calling.' A tone sounded.

'Ahm, er, hello, my name is Fareeda and I've been given your card by a friend who has seen you in the past. Um, I would like to talk to you about counselling. Can you call me, please ...'. Fareeda gave her number and signed off with a 'thank you', and 'I hope to hear from you soon'. She hung up. She realised her heart was thumping. It felt good to have made that call, like she had climbed over some kind of hurdle in doing so. She wondered how long she would have to wait.

It was later that evening that her call was returned. Carla had picked up the message on her return from her afternoon counselling session at a GP surgery. She had spaces for private clients whom she saw at home.

'Hello, is that Fareeda? This is Carla returning your call.'

'Oh yes, hello. Thanks for calling back so soon.'

Carla noted the accent but couldn't quite place it. 'That's OK. How can I help?'

'Well, you've been recommended to me and I need someone to talk to about problems I'm having with my son.'

'Mhmm. Have you had counselling before?'

'No.'

'OK, well, what I would usually suggest is that we meet up for an initial session to discuss what you are looking for from counselling, and I can explain how I work and we can see whether we feel we can work together. I can answer any questions you might have. There is no charge for that introductory session and I suggest about half an hour, and then we decide where we want to go from there.'

Fareeda asked about fees and how often they would need to meet. Carla confirmed her fee and indicated that frequency of sessions was something they would negotiate. They agreed to meet up the following Wednesday in the afternoon. This suited Fareeda as it was her day off. She worked four days a week. She was a team leader at an insurance company. She really valued this. It helped to put more money into the family and was important for her. She also liked her work, the challenge of each day, managing staff and problem solving. She liked to problem solve, but she felt she was facing problems with her elder son that she had no answers to. Fareeda had not worked for periods when the children were younger, but now she appreciated the opportunity of being out of the house, although she was very aware of Ali being in her thoughts.

She also felt guilty as well, wondering whether she was giving up on her family in some way, and whether it was God's will that she made this choice. The tension between what she felt she needed to do, and the question of what she was meant to do, was a constant one.

On a practical level, the job was also important for her because whilst Ali had worked, he didn't contribute much. He tended not to hold jobs down for long. He hadn't really engaged at school, seemed to lose interest in his early teens around the time that Fareeda believed his mood problems to have begun to develop, although he'd been withdrawn for a while before then. Just recently, Ali had begun to spend more time at home, in his room, cutting himself off from people, only going out occasionally in the evening. It had contributed to the tension at home and her own sense of helplessness.

Introductory meeting with the counsellor

Fareeda had rung the doorbell and was waiting for an answer. It was quite a busy street and she was glad that the driveway had room for her to park. Carla had indicated that roadside parking couldn't be guaranteed, but that she could park in the driveway. It wasn't a big house, but there was space for two cars. She waited on the step. A few moments later and the door opened.

Carla saw a dark-skinned woman dressed in a light-coloured suit. 'Hello, you must be Fareeda. I'm Carla. Please come in.'

'Thank you.' Fareeda entered and waited for Carla to close the door.

'Find your way here OK?'

'Yes. I don't live too far away. I know the area quite well. I've parked in the drive – hope I'm not going to be in anyone's way.'

'No problem. Come on through.' Carla led the way to the counselling room, which was a little way along the hall on the right. It was a small room, with two comfortable-looking high-back chairs, a small table, a kind of primrose-yellow emulsion on the walls and a light blue carpet. The curtains matched the colour scheme.

Fareeda took off her coat.

'Here, let me hang this up for you.' Carla took Fareeda's coat and hung it on the peg on the back of the door.

'Thank you. Where should I sit?'

'Wherever you like, whichever appeals.'

Fareeda chose the seat closest to the door. She hadn't thought about it in that way, she just instinctively chose it.

'Does that feel comfortable; I'm not too close or distant?'

'No, that's fine. Thank you.' At some level Fareeda was grateful that Carla was taking the trouble to check this out, and also how she had taken her coat to hang it up. Little things that conveyed a sense of caring and attention, and yet they could mean so much. There seemed to be an intention to care and attend to detail.

'So, where would you like to begin? Do you have any particular questions?'

'Well, I'm wondering how counselling can help me. And you say that you are a "person-centred" counsellor, and I don't know what that means.'

'OK. Well, it's a particular approach to counselling. Let me say a little bit about what it means.'

Fareeda nodded. She sat back in the chair a little. The focus was off her, which helped her relax.

'Counselling, for me, is about offering someone space in which to explore themselves and become more self-aware. I hope that if we decide to work together we can create a trusting environment here in which you will feel increasingly able to be open with yourself, and with me, about what you are experiencing. The person-centred approach is more to do with creating a healthy, therapeutic relationship and for the client to then adjust to that experience, perhaps thereby questioning themselves, but that is something to emerge as and when it happens.'

Fareeda was listening. She liked the idea of space and of trust. She felt good about Carla, the way she spoke, the fact that she seemed quite relaxed and yet had a kind of professional manner as well. But she also felt that reluctance to expose not only herself, but also family issues to a stranger. Her family were Muslim and her experience had been very much that you kept problems within the family, that kin would pull together and do what was necessary to help each other. However, she had adjusted to a different way of life, to some degree, and with only her sister in England she couldn't turn to family in the same way, particularly as she didn't find her sister able to respond in the way that she would have liked. Nevertheless, she regularly said prayers, and read passages from the Koran most days, seeking guidance and direction as to how she should live her life. She had her beliefs, which she was comfortable with. Family was an important part of the Muslim tradition and this had certainly made a strong impression upon her. Chris, however, didn't have that same focus. She put it down to his own cultural background and experience. And perhaps his being an only child had contributed to it as well.

There had been a sense of family, at least, it had seemed more present in the past, but things had changed, and Chris wasn't as she had hoped and expected him to be. She was also aware that her generation was probably not the same as the previous generation, and that for her sons things were different again.

She listened to what Carla had said but was unclear about something. 'What do you mean by a "healthy, therapeutic relationship"?'

'That's really at the heart of it. For me it is about my being able to really listen and hear you – the two are not the same. I want to feel affected by what you want to bring to counselling, and I want to feel able to be honest and open in my responses with you. We call it congruence, but that can sound a bit like jargon. I want to be genuine, honest, transparent, if you like, so the therapeutic relationship we create is two people being genuinely present and increasingly free to be themselves with each other.'

Fareeda nodded again, 'That sounds quite a challenge, to be really open with a, well ...,' she hesitated slightly before continuing, 'with a stranger.' Her thoughts were partly around the sense of 'stranger' but again still with that sense of it being somebody outside of her faith.

Carla nodded, 'And it is unlikely to happen immediately. Trust has to be earned. But my hope is that you will find yourself increasingly able to talk about the difficult areas of your life and your experience – but only if that is what you want to do. For me, therapy is about helping a person become themselves, become more able to freely move around within their personhood, to in effect be more fluid and less fixed in attitude or in particular behaviours and reactions, many of which we may have learned from others rather than being direct expressions of our own essential nature, or that are our own freely chosen way of being.'

Carla is in information mode and has not responded empathically to Fareeda's comment about how challenging it would be for her to be open with a stranger. This is acceptable in the context of an introductory session, perhaps; although an opportunity has passed for Carla to in effect demonstrate her sensitivity and responsiveness to Fareeda. Sometimes in a first contact session like this, the power and nature of the person-centred approach can be best conveyed by its application than by talking about it.

Carla mentions the notion of a person becoming more fluid and less fixed. This is drawn from Rogers' comments concerning his definition of 'Seven stages of process' (1961, pp. 132–59), 'by which the individual changes from fixity to flowingness, from a point nearer the rigid end of the continuum to a point nearer the "in-motion" end of the continuum' (1961, pp. 132). So, for instance, the first stage he defines in the following terms. That 'there is an unwillingness to communicate self. Communication is only about externals' and that 'feelings and personal meanings are neither recognized nor owned'. He suggests that at this stage the client regards 'personal constructs' as 'extremely rigid' and that 'close and communicative relationships are ... dangerous'. He further suggests that the client does not perceive or recognise problems; 'there is no desire to change' and 'there is much blockage of internal communication'.

In contrast, at stage seven, Rogers emphasises the following, that 'new feelings are experienced with immediacy and richness of detail', and 'the experience of such feelings is used as a clear referrent', and that 'there is a growing and continuing sense of acceptant ownership of these changing feelings, a basic trust in his own process'. He adds that experiencing almost completely loses 'its structure-bound aspects and becomes process experiencing – that is, the situation is experienced and interpreted in its newness, not as the past'. At this stage as well, 'the self becomes increasingly simply the subjective and reflexive awareness of experiencing', with the self 'much less frequently a perceived object, and much more frequently something confidently felt in the process', and 'personal constructs are tentatively reformulated, to be validated against further experience, but even then, to be held loosely'. Finally, he points out how at this stage 'internal communication is clear with feelings and symbols well matched, with fresh terms for new feelings' and that there is 'the experiencing of effective choice of new ways of being' (Rogers, 1961, pp. 151–4).

'More fluid. Hmm. That makes sense. I feel quite stuck at times and whilst that's OK in a sense because I do what I do because it's important to me, there are times when I experience a wish to be different, but that makes me feel so guilty.' Fareeda thought of how she felt she should accept things as Allah had created them, and also thought of Ali and how she so wanted to be there for him and to help him, how much of her life had become devoted to being there when he needed her, and yet now and then she did wish things were different for herself. But she could also feel so bad when she had those thoughts and feelings. They really upset her. She was a mother and it was clear to her that a mother must put her children first. It was what she believed and the idea that she could feel different to that troubled her greatly. Made her feel she wasn't being a good enough mum.

'Hmm, want to be different but it leaves you feeling so guilty.'

> Carla now demonstrates her empathy, her response not being a kind of deliberate attempt to demonstrate being person-centred, but rather a natural response by a person-centred counsellor to what she had heard Fareeda say.

Carla did not in her own mind fully differentiate an introductory session from the actual process of counselling. As far as she was concerned they overlapped, although introductory sessions, in her experience, could become more question and answer. What she wanted to try and ensure was that if that was the case it did not set up some kind of expectation in Fareeda that that would be how the counselling sessions would be.

It felt good to Fareeda to feel heard. She'd never said anything about those thoughts and her guilt before. It had just come out and she had immediately felt partly relieved but also suddenly very unsure of herself, feeling that she would be judged for saying such a terrible thing. This sense of feeling judged was something that was very real to her. Her sister in particular seemed to leave her feeling judged, and yet Carla did not sound judging. The way she had responded somehow seemed quite accepting of what she had said. And that puzzled her. It really did not match her expectation.

Fareeda realised she was nodding in response to Carla. Carla, meanwhile, had noted not so much the nodding, but more the fact that Fareeda had immediately looked down after what she had said. She wasn't sure, but it felt to her like Fareeda was maybe embarrassed, certainly that she was uncomfortable. She was unsure as to whether it was more of a cultural reaction – she well appreciated that the maintenance of constant eye-contact was not culturally acceptable to everyone.

Carla had a moment to decide on how to respond. She checked her reaction for what felt to her to be the most pressing response. She realised she wanted to ask if what she had said was making Fareeda uncomfortable. Yes, it seemed right to check that out, and maybe it would also contribute to moving their relationship along, showing her sensitivity to Fareeda's body language.

> It can be helpful to respond to body language. However, excessive responding to body language early on in a new relational encounter can be experienced as quite threatening to a client. It can raise their awareness of their incongruence, for instance, or force into the open discomforts that psychologically they still need to protect themselves from. Empathic responding to body language needs, in my opinion, to be introduced gradually as part of the process of developing trust and openness within the therapeutic context.

'I have the sense that it is quite uncomfortable for you to acknowledge that.'

Fareeda nodded again. She continued to look down.

Carla didn't want the introductory session to develop into a therapeutic encounter, although she recognised that it was not in keeping with the person-centred approach to necessarily keep the two apart. The reality was that from first contact a relationship-building process was underway. Fareeda was forming impressions about her, as she was forming impressions about Fareeda.

Carla waited a few more moments. She felt huge compassion for Fareeda. It suddenly came upon her as she watched her sitting there, head down, contemplating feelings that were so uncomfortable for her. She was also aware of not yet really knowing exactly what Fareeda needed to talk about, what the problems were that she was having with her son, and why they had reached a point now that she was seeking counselling, or what she hoped to gain from a counselling relationship. However, she also appreciated the importance of allowing Fareeda to disclose things at her own pace and in her own way. For the present she had communicated discomfort and guilt in connection with wanting to be different.

Fareeda was taking a deep breath. She was in the process of pushing her feelings aside. She was in the habit of doing this and she really didn't want the awkward feeling that was now present for her to continue any longer. Whilst it felt good that Carla was there listening, it also felt very strange and she wasn't sure what to make of it. She wondered whether this English woman could really understand her difficulties, and her cultural and religious background. She looked up and tried to take in what she saw. Slim, probably late thirties, dark hair, a kind face. But would she, could she, really understand? Could she really help? And what of her son's problems. Would she understand those and the effect it had on her?

'You look to me as though you have lots of questions, and I am aware that we only have so much time today. I don't want to hurry you but I also want to try and ensure you have the answers to any questions you might want to ask related to counselling.' Carla was genuine in what she said. She didn't want Fareeda to leave feeling she had not had a chance to ask what she needed to ask. She also was aware that sometimes, in the stress of the moment, questions were forgotten, or might come to mind after the session.

Fareeda nodded. It helped having someone ask questions rather than leave her to say things herself. 'I guess I still don't really know what I am looking for. I know things aren't good for me at the moment. The idea of coming and talking to someone really appealed.' Carla noted the past tense and wondered whether Fareeda was changing her mind. She felt OK with that so long as it wasn't the result of how she had been so far, or something she had said that was making it more difficult for Fareeda. She could not be sure how Fareeda was interpreting her experience, so she sought to empathise.

'Mhmm, someone to talk to but now not so sure.'

'No, I-I know I want that, but, well, I guess I want to know whether you have any experience of the kind of situation I am in.'

'Mhmm, important to be sure that I can really appreciate what you want to tell me.'

'And there's my culture and religion. I am a Muslim and, well, not being born and brought up in this country, there are a lot of differences. In a way I was lucky, my parents were quite open about other religions although they didn't accept my marrying Chris at first. But they had been encouraging of me to travel here, especially with my sister already in this country. Islam was important to both my parents, and it was very much the way of life for my family. It can be quite a struggle at times to connect to the culture here in England, and at other times I feel quite accepting of it.'

'Sounds like you feel split between Islamic culture and the culture in England?'

Fareeda nodded. Yes, that was how it felt at times, and yet at other times she then felt as though she had integrated to quite a large extent. But that sense of difference was always with her, and she found herself looking at Carla and wondering whether she appreciated this. 'So, I wonder, can you understand what it is like for me?'

'I appreciate what you are saying. I have only worked with a couple of Muslim women and with a few people from different cultures and ethnic backgrounds to my own, but I also want to say something about how this may not necessarily make me a better counsellor for you. Sometimes hearing other people having similarities to a client can leave a counsellor making assumptions, and I want to hear what *you* experience, *your* take on things, and in a way I want that to be clear and fresh. I do not know a great deal about Islam, but I do want to understand what it means to you and what part it plays in your life and your need to seek counselling at this time.' Carla was aware that her comments flowed quite freely, there was no sensation of feeling a need to choose her words carefully. She felt good about that, sensing that what she was saying was genuinely emerging out of her own experience of herself as she sat with Fareeda.

Fareeda listened to what Carla had to say. It felt good that Carla seemed to want to listen, and she could see what she meant about making assumptions. She also had the thought that maybe this would be an opportunity for Carla to learn a little about what life was like being a Muslim woman in England. Perhaps it would help Carla to help others. Whilst she knew that she didn't want someone telling her what to do in the sense of what the Koran would tell her, there was also a part of her that did want that as well. It was all part of her current confusion. Who should she turn to? Who could give her guidance and advice? Was even being here a statement of her diminished faith in Allah? Her friend had really been quite insistent about how helpful Carla had been for her. Her friend was not a Muslim, but she was someone that she respected and felt sure was sincere in suggesting that Carla could help her.

'Thanks for that. I do feel you want to understand.' Fareeda nodded to herself. 'I know I'll want to talk about these things at some point, but not just now. They're important, they will come up, they're who I am.'

'I want to say in response to what you are saying that I welcome that. I know that I will feel enriched by it and it fills me with anticipation for the therapeutic process we may share.' Again, Carla was being genuine. She was experiencing a rush of anticipation. She was going to learn from this encounter with Fareeda, and whilst she knew she must guard against this becoming an agenda for her, nevertheless, the thought of exploring with Fareeda what her religion meant to her, and the dilemma she was experiencing within a religious context, did stimulate a sense of feeling attracted to work with her.

'The other side to all of this is my son, Ali, who, well, I think has problems and it is this that I am struggling with. How best to cope.'

'Coping with Ali's problems are proving to be a real struggle for you?'

Fareeda nodded. She didn't often talk about Ali, and her heart had begun to thump a little. 'Since his early teens he has, I don't know, acted strangely, been very up and down, sometimes outgoing, sometimes he seems to disappear inside himself. I think it's some kind of depression, but I don't know. But it doesn't feel right. And he's been seen but it's only ever put down to "teenage difficulties". It's more than that. I just wish someone was able to help him.' She took a deep breath and sighed, and felt the tears welling up in her eyes.

> The person-centred counsellor won't be thinking about diagnosis. They will want to concentrate on maintaining the therapeutic conditions to allow the client to explore her concerns and to feel those concerns being heard. In this instance, it could be that Ali is struggling with teenage adjustments, but there could be factors that might carry a mental health diagnosis. People do not generally want to hear a diagnosis; there is so much stigma attached, a parent will simply want help for their child to take away the problem behaviours that have emerged.

'So there are two areas – issues linked to being a Muslim woman, as well as coping with Ali's difficulties and the struggle to get him some help.' Carla summed up both the issues.

'And they overlap, of course.'

Carla nodded. 'Yes, it would be false to try and separate them out.'

Fareeda took another deep breath as she thought to herself, yes, they don't just overlap, they're absolutely entwined. How does Allah want me to be? She sighed again.

'So, I really want to have some space to talk it through, unload, get things off my chest, make sense of it all – if I can. I have friends but I don't want to keep burdening them with my troubles. It feels like my marriage may be breaking up over it and, well, I need to, I don't know ...'

'Need to ...?' Carla held the question open, inviting Fareeda to continue if she wanted to. She appreciated how difficult it could be sometimes for people to voice their needs, or even have an appreciation of exactly what their needs were.

Fareeda felt the response immediately, she needed to have a break, get some peace, get away, but she knew that these were things she shouldn't do as well. She was a mother, she had responsibilities and duties. She had been blessed with two wonderful sons. Yes, Ali was a problem to her, and it was her responsibility to care for him. She loved Ali, but sometimes ... sometimes he could be so demanding. She felt tears in her eyes again as she thought these things.

Carla noticed her eyes welling up. 'These are sensitive issues, Fareeda, take your time, say what you want to say when you want to say it.'

Fareeda nodded and took out a tissue to dab at her eyes. 'I'm sorry.'

'It's not easy to have these kinds of feelings and it's OK for them to bubble out.'

'It doesn't feel OK to me. I want them to go away.' She paused, 'But then I don't as well, not really. It's all part of everything. I love my son, and I wouldn't want to be without him, but there are times when I just want to have space between us, but I can't really have that, not really. He just isn't safe sometimes. When he goes, well, whether he's depressed or, I don't know, he's just so difficult to be with sometimes, like he's in another world, and I still have to be there for him.' Fareeda was staring at the wall, her eyes lowered slightly as she spoke. How she had struggled, and how difficult it had been in the family. She thought of Adam as well, he'd not had it easy, probably didn't get the attention from her that he needed. She tried, but . . . Her thoughts returned to Ali, 'He's not seeing anyone at the moment, but I think he needs to be re-assessed.'

'So, Ali was seeing someone for his difficulties but that has ended.'

'There was some family therapy and things eased and he was discharged.'

'OK, so things eased and he was discharged.'

'He drinks some of the time. I think he's also using drugs. Not sure what. He doesn't say much about that. I know he's said that it helps, makes him feel better sometimes, but I think it also makes it worse. I don't know what the real problem is.'

'So, the problem is with his mood, his behaviour and there seems to be a link to drugs, and maybe alcohol, and it really places a lot of demand on you, as you say, you feel that you still have to be there for him.'

'I can't not be there. He's 19 now. My other son, Adam, is younger, and he seems to spend more time with his father. He doesn't seem to have a lot of respect for his brother. They never really have seemed to be close but, well, they've drifted further apart now. Ali spends more time on his own. Adam spends time with his father – at least they are pretty close. It's really splitting us all apart.'

'So there is a lot of stress within the family then. And you are left to cope with Ali. And that feels like it is becoming overwhelming?'

Fareeda nodded. The constant uncertainty as to how he was and what would happen next. Would he be safe? She wished he had more support. In many ways she wished he was the one coming for counselling, but she knew that he wouldn't be interested. She had mentioned it but his response had been that he knew what his problems were and talking to someone wouldn't make any difference. She felt sure that medication wasn't the answer. He didn't see his psychiatrist at the moment, the GP saw him occasionally, but if things became particularly difficult he could be referred back for a new assessment, although she understood that now it would be to adult services and not to the Child and Adolescent Unit where he had been seen in the past. But it seemed to her that when his drinking had become more problematic they had seemed less tolerant of him. She appreciated how stressful it must be for them to work with people, but she also knew how exasperated she had been at times over the years, feeling fobbed off with reasons why he couldn't be offered more care or support. The times that she had begged them to take him in, but was told that he was only worse 'because he was drinking, and they weren't funded to give beds to people who drank too much'.

'Sometimes I just feel like I am having to battle with everyone and I want to run away. And I can't, and I mustn't.'

'Can seem too much, battling with everyone. And, yes, you'd like to run away but can't and mustn't. Battling with everyone and with yourself.'

'It feels like that, like I'm a battleground. And, oh I don't know ...' Another deep breath. 'I have to keep going, somehow. I get strength from my religion. I pray a lot.'

'And I guess that prayer is important and helps?'

'Yes, it is.'

Carla had noticed that time was nearly up. She needed to mention this and draw the session to a close and decide what she could offer.

'Fareeda, time will soon be up and, well, I know I feel good about working with you. I do have a sense of your struggle and really would like to offer you the therapeutic space to, well, use in whatever way you need to.'

'Thanks. I feel like I've said more than I normally would, although I have been silent as well. It's not easy talking about these things. There is so much in my head, so much going round and round, and it never seems to stop.'

Carla nodded, 'And maybe you can find ways of stopping it. I can't guarantee anything. For me, that's how it is with counselling. But I do trust people's ability to find resources within themselves to find new ways of coping with difficult situations. I believe that therapeutic counselling can help to unlock these for people. Though to try and foretell what they will be and how they will work out, to be honest, I don't know. But I am certainly willing to offer you a counselling space here, and we can discuss how often you would want to come along if it is something that you feel will be helpful for you.'

'I do want to come along. I feel a bit hesitant as I am not sure how it will be, but I do need to talk and you have listened today and I really appreciate that. I know you can't change my life, change my circumstances. I guess whilst I'd like things to be different, I know you can't change things. I have to find my own way, but it has been good to talk, even though it has not been easy.'

They continued the discussion, agreeing to meet up initially on a weekly basis and then review this in about six weeks if Fareeda felt that would be useful.

As Fareeda left, Carla returned to the counselling room to reflect on this first encounter. Yes, she did feel good about the prospect of working with Fareeda. She felt herself tight-lipped as she contemplated what her new client had faced and was still having to cope with – broken marriage, younger teenage son now spending more and more time with his father, older son with a mental health problem which Fareeda clearly had had to deal with for a number of years, struggling to get the kind of service that she felt her son needed. And alcohol and other drugs as well.

She knew herself how few Child and Adolescent Mental Health Services (CAMHS) were geared up to work with people using substances as well as having a mental health diagnosis. She shook her head, acknowledging to herself how important such a service was with more and more young people using substances and needing effective treatment – including counselling – to help them resolve life problems and reduce any developing dependence they may have on substances. She knew how widespread alcohol and cannabis use was amongst young people. It was a big problem and she often felt despair that services were not yet being funded to be geared up to respond to the more complex mental health needs of young substance users.

Summary

Fareeda contacts Carla after being recommended to her by a friend. She meets up with her for an introductory session. Fareeda is not sure exactly what she is looking for, but it is linked to her relationship with one of her two sons, Ali. Carla briefly describes her way of working. Fareeda discloses that she is a Muslim and that Ali, her eldest son, seems at times to be depressed, and also to evidence difficult behaviours, although she has not really defined what these are. He has certainly been difficult to cope with and his condition is putting strain on the family system. They agree to weekly counselling sessions and a review.

Points for discussion

- What factors need to be considered when, as a counsellor, you leave a message on an answer machine for clients, and what should be included in that message?
- From a person-centred perspective, what are the key differences between an introductory session and a first counselling session?
- What other elements do you feel should have been introduced by Carla in this introductory session?
- How would you feel if you were Carla and your new client was Fareeda? Would you feel competent to work with her? How would you deal with any sensed lack of competency?
- How would you describe the person-centred approach to a client for whom the words mean very little? What would you emphasise and why?
- Do you think that Carla found the right balance in her use of therapeutic responses in this session?
- What particular issues might Fareeda's marrying outside of her faith have generated, and how would they be impacting on her, and on her family?
- Write your own notes for this session.

CHAPTER 2

Counselling session 1: Wednesday 18th March – issues of race and culture

Fareeda was glad to have the counselling sessions. She had been giving things a lot of thought since the previous week. Although her apprehension remained, she was more convinced of her need to talk things through and try to ease the tension inside herself. She had felt particularly stressed over the weekend and had gone to see her GP, who was glad she was seeing a counsellor. He suggested that she continue to see Carla but come back to him if she felt she needed to discuss any medication to help her feel a little less anxious and overwhelmed by what was happening.

Her GP – Dr Martin – had been very supportive over the years. He was well acquainted with the difficulties that Ali had and the impact that this had had on the family. In fact, at one point he had referred them to family therapy and this had been helpful – they'd had about six sessions. It had brought them together – Ali was 15 at the time, only a couple of years after Fareeda had started to be concerned about Ali's behaviour and mood swings. It had proved to be a useful forum to air views and attitudes; though Chris hadn't attended them all, and it ended at a time when Ali entered a more stable period. But it hadn't lasted. The bullying that Ali had experienced at school in the past was not revealed by Ali. Referral to the Child and Adolescent Mental Health Services (CAMHS) had followed and it was at that time when it had seemed to Ali's mother that Ali had started smoking cannabis and was using more alcohol. But CAMHS hadn't had anyone in their team who had much experience of this and somehow it never got addressed, not really in any meaningful or therapeutic way. At best he was just told to stop smoking, and ease up on the drinking a bit.

> Some CAMHS teams do include a specialist substance misuse nurse and/or therapist. With the increasing numbers of young people using powerful psychoactive drugs (including cannabis and alcohol) the need for this service within CAMHS is becoming more vital. Another model is for CAMHS staff

to be trained in substance misuse work themselves in order to ensure that this is raised appropriately during assessment and that it is included within the treatment responses that are formulated. However, this does have training implications for CAMHS staff.

Service provision varies around the country, which means that in some areas a young person may have access to advice, information and specialist help geared up to their age, and the complexity of a dual mental health and substance use problem; whereas elsewhere this specialist response is simply not available within Child and Adolescent Mental Health Services .

Fareeda went up to the door and rang the bell. Carla let her in and followed her through to the counselling room.

'So, good to see you again,' Carla smiled, 'I don't want to direct you to talk about anything in particular, this is your time, so, where would you like to begin?'

Fareeda smiled weakly in response. She thought for a moment. As she had come up the path there had been so many things in her head to say, but now, well – now she was aware of feeling very much on the spot and unsure where to start. Should she talk about her week, how she was feeling now, the past, her concerns for the future, Ali, her marriage, her beliefs, consulting her GP? She took a deep breath. She was here to talk about Ali, about her struggle to be the mother she thought she should be, about the strain on the family, that was what she had to talk about. But where to begin? She couldn't remember what she had said the previous week, maybe she should give some history?

'Well, I'm not too sure where to start. Ali's had problems since he was 13 or 14; he's never really sort of settled somehow. Now he's 19, nearly 20. He can be moody, and quite artistic at times. Quite expressive. He plays the guitar and has written some songs. At one point he was thinking of going to art college, but somehow that never happened and he left school at 16 and, well, he's had a few jobs, but again, never really settled. And now he's at home again and, well, he doesn't seem to do much. Just stays in his room – comes out to eat. He's on benefits again, I guess that's something. At least he didn't walk out of his last job, he was made redundant. They cut back on staff, he hadn't been there long. But now he just seems to want to drink and smoke cannabis.' Fareeda felt despairing, wondering if Ali would ever hold down a job. 'It's a real drain having him home. Don't get me wrong, I'd rather he was at home, but, well, sometimes I wonder for how long. Will he ever hold down a job? That last one he really seemed to like, but sometimes I just wonder what his future will be, what our future will be.' Fareeda's voice trailed off as she finished speaking. She knew he couldn't stay at home forever, not the way her husband was, but until Ali left could she cope with him? She wanted to, she hoped she could, but the truth was she wasn't sure. And yet it was surely her duty to look after her son? At times it all seemed too much and she tried not to think about it.

For some people with mental health difficulties it can be hard to get employment. Some say that it is easiest where an employer knows, but they do need to be sensitive to the issues. Fareeda is realistic in her concerns and whilst it is not an issue she dwells on in the forthcoming sessions, it is one that people in her position are likely to raise in therapy. Work, if only for short periods, at least would enable Ali to gain more social experience. But at the moment he seems too unstable, and perhaps losing the last job had more of an effect on him than he has recognised, and perhaps on Fareeda, too, who may have seen him enjoying it and begun to feel that he had found something he could commit himself to for a while.

'Hard to imagine what the future will be ..., for Ali ..., and for you.' Carla stayed with what Fareeda had last said, and she spoke slowly, allowing Fareeda time to connect with her thoughts and feelings.

'And, I-I just don't know what to do.' Fareeda could feel herself becoming emotional as she spoke. She had such vivid images of Ali as a child – happy, outgoing, lots of friends. That had seemed to slowly stop, not immediately Adam was born, but over the next few years. The age gap between them was about six years. They hadn't planned to have another child straight away. When Adam was born Ali seemed happy enough at first, he certainly wasn't moody then, perhaps a little withdrawn, but she'd put that down to the arrival of his brother and adjustments in the family. He'd never really seemed quite such a happy child after Adam was born, she never really understood why. And now, now he seemed a different person and she just did not know what to do with him. 'I know how he can be, he was such a happy child, he really was, but now ...' She shook her head.

'You know how he has been, how he can be, but the reality now is different and, as you say, that sense of just what can you do?'

'I should be able to help him, but we don't talk much. At least before he was getting out, but now, well, now he just seems to stay in most of the time. He doesn't seem to want to do anything other than smoke, and I don't know what to do. I worry about him so much. I can't stop worrying.' Fareeda was rubbing her hands as she spoke, clearly there was so much tension held in her arms and fingers.

'Feels like you are constantly worrying about him.' Carla felt for Fareeda. Her own son had struggled during his teenage years, and had experimented with drugs and had taken a while to get his act together, but he had settled down and was now in a long-term relationship and she no longer needed to worry about him as she had done in the past.

Carla has a similar experience but it is *her* experience and it is important that she does not allow her experience to lead her to make assumptions about how Fareeda is feeling. The person-centred counsellor will need to be on her guard to ensure that her empathy is truly that, it is a genuine hearing of what the client is describing. The risk also is that it can attract a sympathetic edge with the counsellor experiencing a sense of 'I know what you mean, isn't it awful'. So counsellors have to be clear and focused, and sufficiently self-aware in order to recognise the nature and motivation of their own internal reactions to what their clients are describing, particularly when they have had similar experiences.

'He's so up and down, at least, that's how he has been. At the moment, well, he doesn't seem to communicate much at all. He's even lost interest in his music at the moment. He has written poetry as well, and some of the things he has written have been so powerful, so deep and moving, really expressing some of his desperation. But now he seems to just cut himself off from everyone.' Fareeda could see him in her mind so clearly, his eyes seemed at times to have lost their life. He seemed so jaded to her, not the son she had known.

'So, a lot of creativity, self-expression, but that seems to have become lost at the moment.'

'He just seems to want to stay in his room, play computer games, listen to music and smoke, and sleep. He's so withdrawn. I wish he'd see someone again but I'm not sure what help he'd get.'

'Seems like you are concerned enough to think he should see someone.'

'I wish he would. I can only see it getting worse. I just keep asking myself, "What did I do wrong?" "What is wanted of me?" ' She shook her head. 'I know I haven't been as devout a Muslim as maybe I could have been, and perhaps should have been. I wonder sometimes, am I being punished for marrying outside of Islam?' she sighed. 'That doesn't seem right and yet ... Oh, I don't know.' She sighed again. 'Trying to make sense of it just makes me feel worse.'

Carla nodded and felt her lips tighten. Her reaction was one of wanting to say, 'You've done nothing wrong, don't blame yourself', but that was her need to save her client from self-blame, and she knew she did not have enough knowledge of Islamic teachings to question Fareeda's beliefs. She was aware of how Fareeda had spoken of feeling guilty and she knew in herself how much she wished parents would recognise that young people choosing to take drugs isn't necessarily some kind of reflection on them, and she personally didn't see it as a punishment. But that was her view, not her client's. So she sought to maintain her empathy, knowing that by so doing she would leave Fareeda to explore her own thoughts, feelings and reactions, and draw her own conclusions rather than be persuaded to feel different because of her counsellor's agenda.

When someone speaks of how their religious beliefs are shaping them, it is not for the counsellor to question those beliefs. It is possible that a counsellor may, or may not, agree with a particular set of beliefs (religious, political, etc.), but effective therapy requires the counsellor to accept and understand the meaning that these beliefs have for the client.

Fareeda's Islamic faith has shaped her and it is an important part of her life. It offers a code for living, indeed, a system for how to conduct one's life. Can Carla offer warm acceptance of Fareeda and of her beliefs? To feel unable to accept her beliefs as valid and important for Fareeda, and as right for her, would be to step out of a person-centred way of working. The importance of empathising with what is present within Fareeda's frame of reference is vital. Fareeda may not want to have to explain her beliefs, that is not why she has come for counselling.

'That's how it leaves you feeling, wondering whether you did something wrong.'
'I do . . .' Fareeda went quiet. But it wasn't long before another train of thought emerged within her mind. She'd tried to get her son the help he needed, but would anyone really take her seriously? She knew, instinctively, that he had problems. She also felt angry. 'And I get angry as well. I shouldn't perhaps feel this way, but I do. I knew something was wrong years ago, but would anyone listen? Would anyone take this minority ethnic woman seriously? I really felt like no one listened.' It had taken a while for Dr Martin to come round to her way of thinking, but even he hadn't really got very far. 'Yes, the family therapy had seemed to help, at the time, at least it seemed to give everyone a chance to talk and for Ali to communicate some of what he felt. But because he seemed to have improved it didn't go any further and we were discharged. And, well, as I say, it helped a bit but things got worse again.' Fareeda closed her eyes. She could remember vividly one occasion, when Ali had been really withdrawn and just didn't want to know about anyone helping him. It really had been difficult. Not all the sessions had been like that though. But Chris not being there all of the time hadn't helped. They hadn't been able to sustain any changes, they hadn't been able to talk more openly in the family or really try to understand each other better.
'And I want to acknowledge that struggle, Fareeda, and I also want to say as well that I am aware of my whiteness in this relationship and it may be something we need to discuss to clear anything that may hinder our openness. I'm not saying now, but I want to communicate my awareness of this.'

It is important that racial, ethnic and cultural differences are addressed, but is this the right moment for Carla to mention colour differences? It is certainly important for counsellors to understand these issues and to be sensitive to them, and to work through them if and when they arise when working with clients where diversity is an issue. The impact of racism, for instance, can generate an oppression-affected self-concept that must be heard by the counsellor. This may not be easy, particularly where the counsellor themself has developed a self-concept that has within it some element of racial superiority. These are sensitive issues, but they must be faced and openly acknowledged. When a counsellor works with a client from another cultural background, or who has a differently coloured skin, it can – and sometimes does – affect the relationship, whether it is white counsellor–black client, or black counsellor–white client.

What form might this take? Both carry thoughts, feelings, attitudes, shaped from their own experiences, and probable prejudices. The individuals' self-concepts will have been affected by the introjected meanings and values that they will have been exposed to, linked to the colour of their skin, ethnic identity, religious allegiances, or other factors encompassed by diversity.

What is important, if there are issues, is that they are recognised and owned. The person-centred approach emphasises the equalising of power between counsellor and client. Some argue that this is never fully possible, others that it is. For instance, the oppressed client – whatever the reason for their oppression – will find it more difficult to experience equality of power and trust of a counsellor who gives off signals that their attempt to equalise power is not emerging from within their essential nature as a person. The counsellor must have to a significant degree resolved any of their own prejudicial, stereotypical or simply plain ignorant thinking concerning race, culture and oppression. The counsellor must take full responsibility for asking themselves what impact their colour, and the colour of their client, is having on their ability to offer the therapeutic conditions. Where it is seen to have, or is at risk of having, a negative or perhaps we should say counter-therapeutic effect, it must be dealt with in supervision and, where necessary, in therapy as well.

Fareeda was aware that she had felt oppressed many times in her life as a result of her colour and her accent. Although she didn't wear the hijab – she had adopted a Western style of dress – it seemed to her that her difference was sometimes all that people saw, and as a result she was treated differently. It felt like she always seemed to come off second best when there were white people around. It wasn't always obvious, but sometimes it seemed as if it was. Sometimes she wondered if she might have had more training opportunities at work if she had been white. She had now simply accepted it as a fact of life. She didn't like it, but she would brush it aside, fed up with feeling she should fight it. In fact, she wasn't as fully aware of just how much it had and did affect her. It had stunted her self-confidence in some areas of her life, and made her particularly sensitive and reactive to racist attitudes. But she said nothing, she had wanted a quiet life in many ways, except where Ali was concerned, and then she had sought to confront the problems that she experienced when trying to get him help.

'I appreciate you saying that but I don't want to get into that, not here. I know you are white, but I see you as a counsellor. Yes, I guess it may affect what happens, but I hope not.' She felt awkward. Carla's comment had felt as though it didn't seem to fit with what she had been saying. It felt like an intrusion and she felt irritated by it. She didn't voice the irritation.

> So long as it was what she was experiencing, Carla might have responded powerfully to what Fareeda had earlier been saying, along the lines of, 'I take you seriously, Fareeda'. This would need to have been said because it was a genuine experience. The person-centred counsellor does not believe in saying things for effect. Anything said must genuinely reflect an experience, otherwise the words will sound hollow, and rightly so, because in reality they are empty and devoid of genuineness and authenticity.

'OK. Maybe it's my stuff introducing this. I don't want to take you away from what you are telling me.' Carla recognised that it was too late, she already had done just that and she knew that she needed to take this to supervision. In herself she realised she was overcompensating against a societal context in which there were a lot of strong feelings against Muslims, and she wanted to ensure she did nothing to indicate she sided with that, however unwittingly it might be. It wasn't that she wanted to compensate for specific prejudicial thoughts within herself, although her belief that most people carry deep-seated feelings and attitudes rooted in cultural and familial conditioning left her aware that she too may at some level carry attitudes that she would prefer not to own. She recognised that she did need to self-monitor, and be aware of what she experienced and how that shaped what she said.

Carla realised that her response had not been timely or appropriate and she needed to clarify this.

Fareeda was shaking her head. 'No, we need to deal with this. I don't feel comfortable and sitting here now I feel like I want to leave, but I also want to stay as well. Leaving would be a way of just avoiding it. Yes, you're right, we are of different colour and I guess have different beliefs, but I'm not here to talk about them. I'm here to talk about the difficulties with my son, but I'm wondering now whether you can really hear me if you are so aware of our differences of colour and background.' Fareeda was not always so outspoken, but she had fought to be heard for Ali, and it was this part of her nature that was driving her to speak now.

'It's all the tension around at the moment and the conflicts that exist in the world, and what I perceive as often ignorant Western attitudes towards Islam. I don't want to be associated with some of the things I read in the tabloids, or hear in the news. I mean, let me give you an example. Someone is arrested on suspicion of terrorism – the news reports that a Muslim man has been arrested. But when do you ever hear of a man arrested being referred to as a Christian?'

'Maybe you would in Islamic countries.'

Carla hadn't thought of that. 'But it isn't right?'

'No, it isn't right, but it happens.'

'You seem to accept it more than me.'

'I've lived with it. It's how it is. We went through years of reading about black muggers, but rarely read about white muggers. Thankfully that seems to have changed a bit, but it's the same racist attitude. You get used to it.'

'But …' Carla felt angry with Fareeda for just accepting something that she wanted to fight for on her behalf. 'I don't understand, and I'm aware that I'm surprised how I am being with you today because I haven't had this reaction before.'

'Maybe today is the right day for you to feel this way.' For Fareeda there was a deep and underlying trust of the will of Allah, although she knew she lost touch with it sometimes. She felt suddenly quite philosophical as she looked at Carla. Could she be the one to help me? At least she is being open about feelings. And it felt good to Fareeda to engage in this conversation now that it had started, however much of an intrusion it had seemed at the start – it didn't often happen.

'Maybe. Look, I don't know what you are thinking or feeling now given what has just been said. I'm genuinely glad that my feelings have surfaced – I'd rather they were visible than buried. I think I am overcompensating for what is happening in society, and I need to set that aside. Yes, I want to relate to you as Fareeda, a woman, a mother, who is worried about her son,' Carla paused, 'and I want to also acknowledge that there are differences between us as well.'

'Then we must acknowledge all these things.'

Carla was nodding. She was seeing Fareeda suddenly as a very different woman, someone with a great deal of self-assurance, strength and self-composure. 'Yes, you are right. Thank you for that.'

They sat in silence for a few moments. It was Carla who spoke first. 'How do you want to continue? You were talking about your struggle to be taken seriously before I raised the issues of race and cultural difference.'

'I think I raised it. It's just been such a battle over the years to get Ali the help and support I've felt he needed and it seems like I am about to have to do it all over again with his current problems.'

'And that can't be easy to face.'

'No, but it has to be done.' Fareeda was in a different place in herself following the exchange that had just taken place, somehow she felt more secure, a sense of poise as she sat observing Carla. 'Ali needs help and he needs me. But I really can't reach him at the moment. I try, but he just seems so distant. So distant. And he can be so negative about life. I must bring in some of his poetry. I'd like you to read it. Some of it is so depressing – commentaries on life, on events – some of it seems so hopeless. I pray for him and I believe in prayer, but it is not enough. I am so afraid of losing him.' She also knew that she hadn't told her sister, or members of her family, the full story. They knew that he had problems with his mood, and that he had been seeking help, but she had not said anything about his cannabis use, and the alcohol in the past. She felt ashamed about his turning to drugs. She knew her parents would not accept it, that it would upset them, so she chose to say nothing and had persuaded her husband to do the same. As these thoughts arose she felt the poise fading again.

The way that Fareeda spoke felt like such a cry for help. Carla responded empathically, holding her on what she had said, inviting her to engage perhaps more fully with what she was experiencing, or maybe explore it further if that was what she wanted. 'Yes, so afraid of losing him.' Carla wished she could look into Fareeda's eyes, she felt she so wanted to reach out to her, but Fareeda was looking down. Carla knew from experience how much unconditional positive regard and understanding could be communicated through eye contact. But she also appreciated that it was not something that was culturally acceptable to everyone, or a comfortable experience for people who were not used to sustained eye contact.

Interesting to note that Carla's desire to reach out to Fareeda is coinciding with Fareeda's experiencing of her desire to reach out to Ali. It could have been a moment for a congruent comment from Carla regarding her sense of wanting to reach out. It might have enabled Fareeda to voice her inner experience. Would it have been directive for Carla to have commented along the lines of 'I am very aware of a sense of wanting to reach out, and I am wondering if that has meaning for you'?

Fareeda so wanted to reach out to Ali. She sat in silence, so aware of her worries and anxieties, of feeling so helpless and questioning her ability as a mother. She knew he had problems, and he seemed to be getting worse. She was taking a deep breath and her husband, Chris, came to mind, or more particularly, his attitude, which was one of constant irritation and anger. He wanted Ali out of the house. He took the view . . . Oh what was the point dwelling on it? She heard Carla's voice: 'You don't need to talk, but I'm here if you want to.'

Fareeda looked up. 'Yes, I know, thanks. I was miles away. I haven't said much about Chris, my husband. He's, oh what's the point in talking about him . . . ?'

It seemed to Carla that Fareeda may not see the point in saying anything, but that she may have a lot that she might like to say. 'So it may not seem like much point in saying anything, but it sounds like you have a lot you might like to say?'

'He's just so fixed.'

'Fixed?' Carla empathised but in such a way as to invite Fareeda to say more, if she wished to.

Fareeda was angry with Chris, and had become increasingly angry with herself for marrying him. Family was so important, it was such an important part of her culture and of her own upbringing. Yes, Ali was difficult, but she had – they had – a duty to be there for him and to help him. But Chris had given up and she wasn't going to forgive him for that. 'Thinks I've spent too much time running around after him.'

'After Ali?'

'Yes. Says I should let him get on with it, that if he had his way he'd throw him out of the house, that that would wake him up, make him take some responsibility. Seems like he just doesn't want to accept that there is a problem. He was really reluctant to attend the family therapy. He didn't get to all of the sessions, said it was work, but I think he was making excuses. I don't think he wants to face up to the fact that his son has problems. Anyway, he isn't much help. I say to him, go and speak to your son, he needs you, he needs someone to talk to him, but, well, Chris isn't very touchy-feely, you know? They just don't get on. I think he's really disappointed with Ali, but I'm sure he loves him, he just can't – or won't – show it.' Fareeda felt a little guilty speaking about Chris like this but she wasn't saying anything that she did not know or believe. And it did feel good having got it off her chest. She sounded off to her sister, but she tended to want to tell her what to do, rather than just listen.

'So Chris finds it hard to accept that Ali has genuine problems and wants him out of the house, which doesn't seem very helpful to you. And your sister . . .'

'No, and we argue about it. He tells me to let him alone and get a life. I can't.' Fareeda paused, feeling tears welling up. She reached for a tissue and dabbed at her eyes. 'I can't, I have my life, as a mother, Ali's mother. He needs me. I have to try and help him. I have to find a way to help him.'

'He's your son, you're his mother, and helping him is so, so . . . , well, so important to you.'

'I have to find a way to reach him. He's a lovely boy, so creative and so sensitive. I'm sure it's the cannabis that's got to him. I mean, he's smoked it for a while and, well, he's never been as bad as this. He drinks, yes, but I don't think that's the real problem at the moment.'

Carla nodded and was aware that there were different types of cannabis. The marijuana often thought of in relation to the '60s and '70s, whilst still available, is not the same as the skunk cannabis that was now so widely available – she'd read somewhere that it was at least ten and sometimes 15 times stronger than the pot or weed of the '60s, though she'd also read elsewhere that that was an exaggeration and the difference was less. It did seem more hallucinogenic and arguably therefore more likely to trigger psychotic reactions because of the strength of the psychoactive components, particularly among people who may have some natural susceptibility to that kind of experience. She wasn't sure how helpful it would be to mention this to Fareeda, it might just add to her worries. But it might also add to her sense of urgency to do something about it. Carla chose to share her knowledge, it was something she knew and, as was often the case in this kind of situation, she would weigh up whether she could justify not saying anything if she withheld what she knew.

The person-centred counsellor does not take on an expert role towards the client. Theoretically, the client is the expert on her situation. She knows best what she is experiencing, what her anxieties are. Her own internal processes are essentially trustworthy and do not need an external expert to direct them. However, this is not an occasion in which the counsellor is trying to show expertise towards the client's process. This is factual information relevant to the client's situation. Of course, if the client was discussing moving house and worrying about what kind of mortgage to take out, then the counsellor would be unlikely to share her opinion or experience, as this would risk directing the client towards a particular course of action, and

> would introduce an external 'locus of evaluation' which would cut across the therapeutic process which is towards enabling the client to cultivate and strengthen their internal 'locus of evaluation'. So, in this case where the information that Carla has is directly relevant to Fareeda's son's well-being and mental health, Carla takes the view that she could not defend not sharing her knowledge; that by withholding it it would diminish her unconditional positive regard towards Fareeda and her seeking to be genuinely present and authentic in their relationship.

'I don't know if this is helpful, but there are different types of cannabis. There is a type that has been introduced in recent years called 'skunk' cannabis, said by some to be much stronger than what we know more as marijuana, weed, pot.'

'I didn't know. So, you mean, Ali might be smoking something stronger?'

'Well, I don't know, but I am aware of this but I don't know much more than that.'

'I need to know more. Where can I find out?'

'Local drug agencies – there are a couple in the area. Numbers are in the *Yellow Pages*, I think. There is also a national drugs helpline for young people, "Talk to Frank"'*. I don't know the number, though.'

'Thanks for that. I mean, I'm not sure that I wanted to know that, but I'm glad I do. Maybe Ali doesn't realise. Maybe I can, I don't know, try and help him to understand.'

'Mhmm. Talk to the agencies. I think one of them specialises in working with young people. It's unfortunately a growth area these days, but, well, I'm sure they can give you the information you want, and maybe they'll have leaflets you can give to Ali as well.'

'I feel more anxious but also glad I have a sense that there is something I can do. You're right. I need to get some facts.' Fareeda paused and frowned, 'And they're making cannabis a less serious drug, aren't they?'

Carla nodded.

'And yet it's now stronger than it was?'

Carla nodded again. 'That seems to be a possibility.' There wasn't much more to say really. She didn't want to get caught up in a discussion over the arguments for and against changing the classification related to cannabis use.

'Are we going mad?'

'That how it seems?'

'And so my son is now less likely to be, what, charged for using cannabis, or get less of a punishment, yet what he's using is probably now stronger than it would have been a few years back when the laws were tougher?' Fareeda paused, she was now maintaining steady eye contact. 'I'd write to my MP except that I wouldn't trust him to not pass the details on to the police.'

---

*Talk to Frank. A national, free and confidential drugs information and advice service for young people – 24 hours a day. Tel: 0800 776600. Website: www.talktofrank.com, and email: frank@talktofrank.com, and if you are deaf, textphone: 0800 917 8765.

'Well, that's the law as I understand it too.' Carla sought to focus on being empathic towards Fareeda, whose tone of voice was clearly communicating a sense of outrage. 'You sound pretty outraged by it.'

'Yes, I am. I could knock a few heads together.' Fareeda's words sounded humorous but there was no humour intended. Carla did not smile but maintained her own serious expression.

'You sound strong, Fareeda, and serious.'

'I suppose I am. Strong, that is. I can be about some things, you know.'

'I don't doubt it, and one of those is Ali, yes, and getting heard and getting his needs met.' Carla wasn't sure whether she was directing Fareeda back to what she had said before, but somehow it just felt like the most natural response to make, bringing things together, in a way drawing together some of the threads of the session. As she finished speaking, Carla glanced at the clock. Yes, time passing and the session only had about five minutes to run. She mentioned this, wanting to be sure that Fareeda could work within the time available.

'Yes, I know. Funny, what we were just talking about has fired me up, somehow. I needed that. I'm going to contact those agencies and get the information and see what advice they can give me. I don't care what Chris thinks. Ali's my son and I'm his mother, and I'm not giving up on him.'

'That sounds very clear to me, Fareeda. You're not giving up on him.'

'Thanks for the session. Let me pay you.' Fareeda handed over a cheque for the agreed fee.

'Thanks. So, I hope the session has been helpful and, well, I know we got a bit bogged down ...' Carla was back to thinking about the difficulties they had had earlier in the session, 'but maybe that helped in some way. I feel more connected with you now.'

'I do, too. Thanks for listening. I do feel heard. And thanks for telling me about the, what was it, "skunk"? What a horrible name.'

'I think it's because of the smell.'

'I have noticed the odour in his bedroom has been a bit strong. I put it down to teenage stuff, you know, hormones and the like. Maybe it isn't that.'

'Get some advice and, well, good luck.' Carla paused. 'You intend to continue with the counselling?'

Fareeda nodded. 'Yes, this is for me, my space, my time.'

'We agreed weekly, yes?'

Fareeda nodded.

'So, same time next week OK, and I'll keep that time open for you weekly for now, yes?'

'Yes please. Thanks.'

The session ended. Fareeda left with an awareness that whilst she felt a little stronger, she was also aware that her anxiety as to what Ali was doing had increased. But she was determined to get the facts for herself. Yes, she felt good about the counselling. It had felt awkward at times, but that seemed to have passed. She felt glad that she had generally been quite composed. She didn't want to get in a state and then have to cope with it afterwards. No, she was glad that Carla had been recommended to her. She felt that they would get along.

She knew her problems went beyond Ali, but how much she would talk about it, she did not know. She felt so split, sometimes, so torn between wanting the best for her son and wanting to somehow try and hold on to her marriage. And yet, the latter wasn't good, and she had turned to the Koran for guidance. She didn't feel the marriage was over, and she had their younger son, Adam, to think about. He seemed OK, and somehow closer to his dad. She often wondered whether it had been wise to name the children in the way that they had. She wondered what effect it had had. Had it alienated Chris from Ali? She didn't want to think so, she was sure it was simply because of the way Ali had been behaving in recent years. She felt sure Chris loved him, she wanted to believe it.

Carla meanwhile was standing waiting for the kettle to boil. It had been quite a challenging session and she was left with material to discuss at her next supervision session. Was she overcompensating for her own uncomfortable feelings about the way certain people viewed Islam and Muslim people in the West? Was she too sensitive in bringing up the issue herself so soon? She knew she wanted to explore this and it seemed that her supervisor was the first place to start, although she also wondered whether it might be better taken to her next therapy session. She decided to take it to supervision first and then, if it seemed to require further work, then she would take it to therapy.

Summary

The first counselling session brings issues of racial, cultural and religious difference and diversity to the surface for both Fareeda and Carla, and Fareeda's sense that as a foreign woman it has been harder to get help for Ali. Carla is left feeling that her reaction needs processing in supervision, or possibly therapy. Fareeda describes her frustrations in trying to get help for her son, Ali, over the years, how unhelpful her husband is, but how determined she is to try to reach out to Ali, who is spending more and more time isolating himself in his room and using cannabis. Carla mentions that she has read that 'skunk' cannabis is said to be much stronger than the cannabis referred to as marijuana, weed or pot.

Points for discussion

- What was your reaction to Carla's handling of the racial and religious/cultural issues raised in this session? How might it have been handled better?
- Consider your personal reaction to Ali. Is this reaction a pure response to the session, or is it affected by other material from your own life experience?
- What issues would you specifically take to supervision if you were Carla, and how would you raise them?

- Fareeda feels very split in herself. List the factors that have contributed to this that have been highlighted, and extend your thinking beyond what has been disclosed to what else may have contributed to this.
- Critically evaluate the quality of empathy offered by Carla during this session.
- What were the most significant moments during this session?
- Was Carla right to introduce information about cannabis? Whatever your view, can you justify this theoretically?
- Write notes for this session.

CHAPTER 3

Supervision session 1: Friday 20th March – processing issues of race, culture and belief

'I've got a new client, William, and there are some issues I need to address with you.'

William, Carla's supervisor, sat opposite her, stroking his beard as he was wont to do, and smiled a sort of inquisitive smile. She knew how much he loved the quest of self-exploration, the search for greater understanding when it came to how people interacted.

'Tell me more.'

'Fareeda is a mother of two sons. One of them, Ali, has been experiencing mood swings for some while and is now using cannabis and is withdrawing into himself. There's a likelihood that he's self-medicating to feel better. She's trying to support him, feeling guilty for not being a good enough mum, has a husband who doesn't want to know and who thinks the son should be thrown out. She is at times at the end of her tether.'

'Stressful, and what else?' William sensed that there was more to be said.

'There are cultural and religious factors. Fareeda is a Muslim. She draws from the Koran for guidance and, well, it's my reaction that I need to explore here.'

'So, something about how you have reacted to Fareeda because she is a Muslim, or a Muslim woman? Where's the emphasis?'

'No, it's because she is a Muslim and, well, I introduced the fact of our differences and I think it wasn't the right time, but it happened. It has left me really questioning myself as to whether I can really, I mean really, empathise with her in a way that is truly reflective.'

'You mean, you are not sure that your empathy is accurate?'

'What came up was my sense of overcompensating for the attitudes of Western societies towards people who follow the Muslim faith. I don't believe we – that's "we" collectively – the white Christian "we" if you like, I suppose – I don't believe we really accept the Muslim world view. We don't understand and we find it all too easy to look down on this group of people as being somehow inferior, and because they have different beliefs and traditions. And that's wrong and I don't like it and I don't want to be part of it. But I think that – look, let me

give you an example. The issue of racism came up in the session and Fareeda spoke in terms of accepting it as being the norm. And I was angry. I was outraged. I couldn't accept that view. Racism is wrong, as far as I am concerned.'
'Mhmm, I hear you, and I hear the passion. And you speak of overcompensating and not believing your empathy is accurate?'

Carla has talked about 'white Christians', when in fact all religions involve people from all colours, and what she says might also in a sense imply a belief that all Muslims are coloured or black, which is also untrue. It says something about the way she thinks, and William has not picked up on it either. Had he responded to this he might have enabled her to explore and understand her own deep-seated associations between race, religion and colour.

'I don't want to appear to be siding with a view that exists in Western society that is not merely non-accepting of the Islamic faith and the people who follow it, but is actually out and out hostile towards it. I guess I hadn't been put in this position before.' Carla went silent, aware of feelings of unease within herself. She sought to stay with them, knowing from experience how important it was for her to allow what became present to emerge more fully into awareness.
'So, having Fareeda as your client now, in the current social context, is proving . . . , I'm not sure what word to use, but is making it difficult, let's say?'
'I mentioned our colour difference and Fareeda said that yes, she was aware of it but was actually coming to see me because I was a counsellor, and she later expressed doubt whether I could really hear her if I was too busy being aware of cultural or racial differences. I can't remember how she put it, but she was right. That's the problem. Am I too aware of our differences and what that means in the social context, and is it going to get in the way of me actually hearing what she has to say? It is about her relationship with her son and her anger and frustration at feeling he has not received the help she believes he should have had in the past, and how she should cope now that he seems to be using cannabis so heavily. These are not issues of race, these are human issues, but I'm left doubting myself.'
'Like you want to turn it into something other than what Fareeda is bringing?'
'That sounds awful but, yes, I have to admit that I think you're right.' Carla did not like hearing herself say this, but she knew she had to.
'So, what are you trying to prove, Carla, and to whom?'
Carla tightened her lips as she took a deep breath. 'This doesn't feel good, William. I want to . . . No, let me try again. I don't want to appear to be ignorant of difference, colour, religion, and I don't want to . . . I don't want to be associated with some of the societal attitudes that I read about or hear people expressing. I suppose I want to be politically correct, I mean, yes, I do, but I think I can become too aware of that as well.' She paused for a moment or two. William

did not interrupt, he could see Carla was focusing on something within herself. 'I just want to relate to her as a woman under stress, struggling to find a way through life. That's where and how I want to meet her. But I'm not sure that I can, or am. I've got this other agenda in my head. Prove you're not like the others: the racists, those who are just full of ignorant prejudice. I don't want to be seen to be like them.'

'Mhmm, you don't want to be seen to be like them, and it sounds to me as though you are pretty damn sure as well that you don't want Fareeda to see you as one of them.'

Carla was slowly shaking her head and looking down as she responded, 'No, I don't.'

'So you try to make her see you differently, but in so doing you lose your empathy for her, for what she wants to communicate to you.'

Carla was still nodding. She took a deep breath and sighed. 'Yes. My needs are getting in the way of being able to hear her. I'm sure it didn't happen all the time, but it's there, isn't it?'

William nodded.

'How do I resolve it? Do I take it to therapy?'

'Well, it seems to me to be a supervision issue at the current time, but yes, it could be taken to therapy as well, to be explored in a wider context than your specific work with Fareeda. Maybe there are thoughts and feelings you need to air and process. But I think that there is a place for this in supervision so that you can be supported in being an effective counsellor with your client.'

It is a matter of professional judgement to decide whether an issue can be handled in supervision, or whether it requires therapy. How does one make this judgement? It is not easy. In the person-centred approach a major focus of supervision lies in ensuring that the counsellor is able to offer the therapeutic conditions accurately. This is fundamental and can therefore involve a lot of focus on the counsellor and some traditions in counselling might see the person-centred supervisor dealing with issues that they would consider to be topics for therapy. Perhaps the answer lies in the time needed to work on an issue, given that supervision is time for counsellors to reflect on and review their work with a number of clients, or supervisees, and there may simply not be the time – unless extra supervision sessions are agreed to focus specifically on the difficulty that has arisen.

'You don't think I'm being effective?'

'I'm not in the session, what do you think? How do you experience yourself with Fareeda, and, more importantly, how does she experience you?'

'She said she was uncomfortable and wanted to leave, but that she knew that wouldn't solve anything. She then said something that really stayed with me, and you know, makes me feel quite emotional thinking about it.'

William turned his head slightly, raising his eyebrows in a manner that invited Carla to elaborate further on this.

'She said to me, in response to my feeling angry and experiencing my reaction to being with her, she said that "maybe today is the right day for you to feel this way". Which for me means maybe the time was right for my feelings to come out, and probably so that I can address them. The last bit is my interpretation.'

'Mhmm, so maybe it is.' William deliberately left the words in the air and waited for Carla to respond. It wasn't that he wanted to side with Fareeda, he didn't know whether this was the right time, but in a sense he did know because he trusted the inner processes of people and clearly something was happening for Carla and for her, however unsettling, it was timely.

'Maybe.' Carla sat quietly reflecting on what had occurred. Fareeda's words helped her to feel a little calmer as she sat thinking about her reactions. 'Maybe.'

William sat with an attitude of warm acceptance towards Carla. He wanted to support her in her work with Fareeda. He did not doubt the timeliness of what had happened and he did want to help Carla resolve this, or at least contribute to her process. It seemed to him that Carla had been offered a gift but at the time had not seen it as that. He wondered whether to say this, or to wait to see if Carla could see that for herself. He didn't want to project his meaning on to the situation and thereby in some way undermine any meaning that Carla was developing for herself. So he waited a while longer for Carla to continue.

Carla sat with a very clear image of Fareeda in her mind, of her sitting there and being somehow so accepting of her, Carla's, clumsiness. For that was how it now seemed to her. Fareeda's words were still clearly with her. She took a deep breath and was about to speak, but wasn't sure what to say. She stayed silent a little longer. Eventually she managed to draw her thoughts together into a sentence.

'I think that she may have given me something quite precious.'

'Precious?' William sought to empathise but offer an opportunity for greater clarification.

'It's the old story, we get the clients we need at least as much as, hopefully, the clients get the counsellors that they need.'

William nodded. He also believed this to be the case. He was never sure who was necessarily gaining the most from the therapeutic endeavour that was counselling. He knew that he constantly learned about himself through his work with clients. They invariably came bringing issues for him to work on as part of the therapeutic process. 'I would say that we need to be open to receiving the gifts that our clients bring to us.'

'Fareeda is bringing me an opportunity, here; an opportunity to learn, an opportunity to be . . .', Carla smiled, 'the word "humble" comes to mind.'

William nodded. 'Humble. Humility. How do you see that in this context, Carla?'

'I feel humbled, I really do. People like Fareeda – God, that sounds awful saying it like that. But words are so cumbersome sometimes. But, you know, she has had to put up with a lot of shit, a lot of shit, and yet she perseveres and she maintains something in herself, I don't know what it is, but it's something I've seen in other Muslim women. I don't know exactly how to describe it, but there's a kind of... it's like humility but that isn't the word I want. It's like a kind of faith that somehow all will be well. It's like, yes, a deep trust in I guess the will of God, I mean, of Allah. There's like a deep acceptance. And I know I'm generalising here, and I'm sure that not everyone may carry this kind of aura, I suppose, but I have seen it, I have experienced it, and Fareeda has it.' In the moment of saying those last few words Carla was struck by a sense of her own inadequacy. 'And I wish I had it.'

'The thought that is with me is that it is somehow hard for you to accept her deep acceptance.'

Carla nodded, 'And I also know that there are things she does not accept and fights for, and I'm thinking of Ali, her son.'

'Yes. And you can accept that?'

Carla smiled. 'Yes. But you know, that other, deeper acceptance, you know I don't think that is always for real. I think that it can be, but it can also be conditioned, forced on women to develop so that they don't question.' Carla looked surprised to hear herself speak this way. 'You know, I hadn't really thought about it quite like that before, but now, well, I mean, thinking of conditions of worth, the pressure to think of yourself in a certain way in order to be accepted among the faithful. That's an enormous pressure.'

'So there is like "true acceptance" and a "false acceptance", is that what you mean?' William wanted to clarify exactly what Carla was saying. He could appreciate where she was coming from but wanted it to be really clear and visible.

'I don't know, but something like that. I mean, I feel that generally about all religions actually, I'm not really being specific here, though I might sound it.'

'So, given what you have been saying so far about your reaction to working with Fareeda, I'm wondering where this leaves you now?'

'Immediately, the feeling comes to mind that I really want to get to know her, I mean, really get to know her. I don't think I've been doing that. I've been listening but, yes, with my own agenda. I want to hear her. I think something has cleared. Whether it has fully cleared, I'm not so sure, and I may well need to come back to this. And I'll see how the next session goes before deciding whether to take something of this into therapy. I almost want to say that it's between Fareeda and me – well, it's actually between me and myself – sorry, that's probably confusing you. I recently saw an Alan Ayckbourn musical "Me, Myself and I", about different parts of a person. But that's a digression.'

'It's OK, I've seen it, I can appreciate what you mean.'

'And I want to almost keep it where it belongs, where it has arisen. Do you think that's OK? Or am I fooling myself here?'

'How do you feel about sitting with Fareeda now, feeling as you do as a result of our exploration or, if you like, this collaborative enquiry this evening?'

William enables Carla to reflect within the supervision session on the work they have done together, giving her time to assimilate what has occurred and to consider whether anything has changed for her. This can be helpful, enabling the supervisee to acknowledge what has occurred. The person-centred supervisor will want to encourage the supervisee to gain her own insights and to draw her own conclusions as to what has emerged through the supervision process.

'I feel much more at ease with the idea. I think I can be much more present for Fareeda with what she wants to talk about. It's been really helpful airing all of this. It's taken up a large part of the session but it's been important. I'm sure I'll bring her again, but thanks. I really must move on to talk about a couple of other clients.'

'OK, well, I want to say that I appreciate your honesty and openness in bringing this to supervision. Supervision is so dependent on the integrity of the counsellor, of your readiness to self-question and bring difficult issues into this setting. So, thanks. It's thought provoking. I am sure you will be there for, and with, Fareeda when you next see her and I really look forward to hearing how the relationship develops. I feel she is safe in your hands, Carla, and I know you will continue to self-monitor.' William was utterly genuine in what he was saying and this was conveyed to Carla.

'I think it's important to have something of an internal supervisor. But I appreciate hearing what you have just said.'

Without doubt, Fareeda would benefit from the openness and honesty of the supervisory discussion and exploration that had just occurred. Carla moved on to discuss another client.

Counselling session 2: Wednesday 25th March – poetry and an emotional release

Fareeda was a little early and waited outside in her car until her appointment time was due. She walked to the door thoughtfully, and rang the bell. Carla answered and invited her in. After giving her the cheque for the forthcoming session, Fareeda took out a piece of paper from her bag.

'I feel like I want to help you understand something about Ali. He's not been too good this week, withdrawn, even more so. And I took your advice, I did contact the Drug Team and they were really helpful. They said that they would be happy to see him, but that really he needed to want to attend. They sent some information in the post, and I've given it to Ali. He hasn't commented and I haven't followed it up yet. They told me to give him space, not push too much, but try to be consistent with him, and show that I'm acting out of caring about him. So, thanks for that, and I hope to get him along to see someone there. But I realise that may take time.'

'So you've been quite active by the sound of it, and you feel it has been positive but, yes, as you say, it may take time before he comes around to feeling he might need help.'

Carla was aware that she was feeling different to the way that she had the previous week. She was listening to what Fareeda was saying and it felt as though some of the other issues that she had discussed in supervision had melted away. She didn't feel the need to dwell on it but let the observation pass.

'It's been difficult. I find I'm reluctant to go to work some days, and I hurry back to check he's OK. He always is, but, well, I suppose the one thing about the cannabis is that he seems more predictable, at least at the moment. In the past, well, he'd just go off and do things, or go places, get something in his head and act on it. I know that's normal teenage stuff, but he'd get on a train somewhere and travel real distances – like once we got a call from Wales! He'd got on a train because he wanted to be in the mountains. He hadn't paid for the ticket and couldn't get a train back, and didn't have enough money. We had to go and collect him. Things like that. Get it in his head and off he'd go.'

Carla listened and felt for her. She wondered how she would have reacted, and felt sure that once the anger had subsided she'd have wanted to understand why. But it seemed like this kind of thing was normal for Ali, and for his parents to cope with. 'So he could cause you to run around a lot after him?'

Fareeda nodded. 'And that was usually when he was on a high, as I saw it anyway. When he was like that he could do anything – except that he couldn't. It was so difficult to contain him, and then he'd crash down and just withdraw.' Fareeda paused. 'In a way it was a more intense withdrawal than where he is at the moment. It was like he was so caught up in whatever was happening inside himself that he couldn't really engage outside of his world. I don't know.' She sighed. 'Anyway, I brought this along. Something he wrote some while back after he'd had a really low period. It says so much and I often read it and remind myself of something of what happens inside him.'

'It sounds really important to you, really helps you to connect with his inner world.' Carla kept her empathic response simple and focused on the last thing that Fareeda had said, offering her the opportunity to flow with her stream of thinking and feeling and not be drawn back to what she had previously said.

Fareeda nodded. 'I'd read it to you but it makes me sad. Can you read it?'

'If that is what you would like.'

Fareeda nodded again and handed her the piece of paper.

Carla looked at it. At the top of the page was a title: 'Nowhere Left to Run'. She felt herself going silent inside as she began reading. The words were powerful, dramatic.

> Hitting out, violent shout. Storm clouds fill the air.
> Shattered dreams, silent screams, a world without a care.
> You and me, we can see, frustration all around.
> Bottle up this bitter cup beneath a burial mound
> Of frightened eyes, distorted lies, that tell of pains and fears,
> Forever caught as slaves of thoughts, will no one dry my tears?
> I cannot cope without a hope, there's nowhere left to run,
> So standing still upon that hill I face my setting sun.

Carla sat very still as she scanned back over the words again, aware that they really were making an impact upon her. Whatever must Ali have been feeling, and what must Fareeda have thought and felt when she first read it? And what must she feel now, still carrying it with her. There was a date at the bottom of the poem, it had been written three years ago. 'That's powerful. It leaves me feeling very still and quite emotional.' She paused as she looked across at Fareeda, 'And I wonder how it affects you, Fareeda.'

'Tormented. It's not a world I can relate to and yet it's so graphically present somehow in his words.' She swallowed, feeling a surge of emotion. Her throat felt like it was blocked and the tears were welling up in her eyes.

'Mhmm, hard to relate to and yet it is so present in his words.'

Fareeda was looking down and could feel the tears trickling free over her eyelids. She swallowed again. 'I have to help him, Carla, I have to. And all I get is my husband saying he's a waste of space. I-I don't think I can take it anymore.' With that last comment she burst into tears, sobbing away the built-up frustrations and hurt, and the feeling of being so alone in her struggle to help her son. The sobbing continued.

Carla sat with her feelings of compassion for Fareeda. Words of a song came to mind – she couldn't remember who sang it – 'You and me against the world' must feel like that, she thought to herself. Carla had learned to trust these strange promptings or connections within herself when clients were in touch with deep feelings. 'Must feel like it's you and Ali against the world.'

Fareeda nodded, whilst trying to dry her eyes with a tissue. 'Ye-es, ye-es, that's, how, it, feels, sometimes.' The words came out in a broken way, caught between the short breaths that she took amongst her tears.

Carla reached over and touched Fareeda's arm. She felt she needed to make some kind of physical contact – so much of the pain was manifesting at a very physical level – she felt strongly that a physical response would be the most empathic one.

Touching a client is often seen as a difficult area. From a person-centred perspective I would argue that if a client is in distress and the motive for touch is a sincere and genuine reaching out from one person to another, and there is not much likelihood of it being misinterpreted by a client, then frankly, what is the problem? We sometimes need to communicate compassion through touch, or a sense of solidarity, or of reassurance. Yes, there is a risk of a client misinterpreting it. And perhaps there is a need for a 'when in doubt, don't' attitude, but even then, the counsellor must be sure about the origin of their doubt. It could be their own fears or sensitivities obstructing a natural, therapeutic response. Unease around touch, or lack of any unease, both need processing in supervision. The counsellor has to be clear in herself, has to know the true origin of this form of responding. An ability to trust their inner prompting rooted in congruence and self-awareness is vital.

Fareeda felt the contact – it was reassuring. She swallowed and took a deep breath. 'Ohh.'

'Lot of feelings, so much struggle and hurt.'

Fareeda nodded. She closed her eyes as another wave of emotions tore through her. She hadn't cried like this in the longest while, perhaps she had stopped herself, afraid of what would happen. But now she was crying and she felt like she might never stop. Her breathing continued in short, sharp intakes of air. She wanted to get away from the feelings inside herself but she couldn't. She felt Carla squeezing her arm a little more for a moment or two. It drew her momentarily away from herself but immediately she was back in the torrent of emotion that it seemed was overwhelming her.

'Oh God, Oh God.' Fareeda's body jerked as she struggled to breathe. 'Oh God.'

Carla recognised that this cathartic release of emotion needed to happen, it happened to be today, now. She moved closer and knelt down in front of Fareeda, and held her other arm as well.

Fareeda needed more than this contact, but she also felt herself hesitating. She wanted to be held, Oh God how she wanted to be held. And yet, there was a barrier, and it was the fact that Carla was different – different colour, different ethnicity. She wanted to break through that barrier but she could feel herself holding back. She shouldn't do that, she must pull herself together. She needed to maintain her dignity. Another wave of emotion and the barrier was broken, it was like a damn bursting and she put her arms around Carla, continuing to cry, holding her tightly like she felt she never wanted to let her go.

Carla responded by seeking to hold Fareeda in equal measure. Carla had closed her own eyes, feeling the emotion of the moment herself. It was after a few minutes that she felt Fareeda loosening her grip, and she responded in the same manner.

'I'm sorry.'

Carla felt herself shaking her head. 'You needed to let that go, Fareeda, I'm glad to have been here for you.'

Fareeda's breathing was still a little broken, and she still struggled to swallow with the lump she could feel in her throat. 'I just keep thinking back to that poem that sense of him standing there, without hope, no one to dry his tears, no one to dry his tears . . . I tried to be there, Carla, I've tried to be there, and I want to be a good mother. But the thought that I wasn't there to dry his tears . . .' She felt more tears welling up and she tightened her eyes to try and hold them back but they forced their way out and she again felt them, hot and trickling down her cheeks. 'I love him. I know he's done crazy things but he's a good son, he really is, I know he is. I can feel it, call it a mother's instinct, I don't know, but I'm afraid of losing him. I so want to reach out to him, and I want others to reach out to him.'

Carla nodded gently. 'Yes, you want to reach out to him and you do reach out to him. But at the moment he's not able or not wanting to reach back.' Carla wasn't sure whether she should have added the second part of her response. She recognised it as being an attempt to try to ease Fareeda's distress, and that wasn't what she should be doing. And yet it seemed as well that what she had said was probably perfectly true.

'No, he isn't. But I have to keep trying, I can't give up on him, not like Chris. He's a self-centred bastard. He gets so damn moody about it. It's his son, our son, we both need to be there for him but it's only me, only me trying to help and I don't know whether I am being much help.'

'That's a hard place to be, Fareeda, doubting whether you are helping.'

Fareeda had begun to sit back and the two women let go of each other. 'Yes, it is.' She took a deep breath. 'Thank you, I've never felt like that before, and I've never cried like that. Felt like I was crying not just for now, but for a number of years.'

'It gets bottled up.'

'I mustn't let it bottle up like that again. I have to do something. I have to.'

Carla nodded and she was suddenly so very aware of thinking, yes, and you must look after yourself as well. She held the thought and responded to what Fareeda had communicated. 'Yes, you know in yourself that you have to do something.'

Because a therapist experiences something does not mean they should verbalise it. A misunderstanding as to the meaning of congruence is the notion of saying anything and everything that becomes present within the therapist. People might say that this is about being transparent, but in actual fact the first duty of the counsellor, in my view, is to listen, to offer empathic responses to what the client is communicating. If this can be done with an attitude of unconditional warm acceptance for the client, then even better. And where the counsellor is genuine and authentic in their presence, then the likelihood of therapeutic movement in the client is increased further. But counsellors who think their first duty is to communicate whatever they think or feel to the client are a menace. Communication of what becomes present for the counsellor must be relevant to the therapeutic process and emerge from a sense of connection with the client. And even then, there may still be reasons not to communicate, for instance so as not to divert a client away from a focus that they have developed and which clearly it is important for them to continue to explore. Effective person-centred therapy requires self-discipline on the part of the therapist.

'I've got to get him seen by the people at that drug service. Somehow I have to persuade him. It'll only get worse. I have to try, and keep trying.'

'Mhmm, thought of not trying is just . . .'

Fareeda was shaking her head. 'Couldn't do that. He's family. Flesh and blood, my son. I have to help him and I will do. We look after our own.'

Carla nodded and smiled gently. 'That comes from the heart.'

Fareeda nodded. 'You know, I've thought about wearing the hijab. As I've got older, Islam has become more important to me. Something about identity, my identity, who I am. Does that seem strange?'

In fact, and Carla was a little surprised herself, it somehow didn't seem strange at all. 'If someone had said that before I'd have wondered at it, but hearing you speak, and how important Islam is for you as a way of life, no, I don't think it is strange. It sounds like something you need to do for you.' Carla had noticed the emphasis on 'I' in what Fareeda had been saying and so sought to capture this in her response.

'It is. It is a sign, a symbol, and it signifies a change in me. It's like I feel I must return home – not literally to Mauritius, but to the Islamic way of life. I feel like I have wandered afar, but maybe I need to return home. I'm not a Western person, not really. I've maybe fooled myself, but I think I've known for a while that it isn't me, not really.'

The session continued but with less intensity. Fareeda felt drained and really struggled to focus on much else. She said at one point that she felt like she just wanted to sit quietly. Carla offered her a cup of tea, which Fareeda accepted. It felt good to just take a bit of time to quietly come back together. She had really wondered whether the crying would ever stop, the emotions, the hurt had just felt like it might go on forever. As she sat and sipped her tea she looked down at the poem that had been put on the small table between them. She swallowed, her throat was feeling easier now.

'Thanks for being here, Carla, we've hardly spent much time together but some-how I feel like I've made a connection.' She thought of how she had felt herself blocked from holding Carla, and how that had dissolved under the force of emotion. She decided not to say anything about it. She was a little bit ashamed and yet it also felt important for her to take away from the session.

Carla was quite unaware of the internal struggle that had occurred within Fareeda. She knew that she felt much closer, felt that the human experience between them just transcended differences.

The session drew to a close and Fareeda left, feeling a little more grounded after having taken time to sit quietly and also feeling a little lighter in some way as a result of letting go of so much emotion.

It was later, after the session, that Carla had time to reflect on her sense of the importance of sharing those common human experiences that transcend differences. Human feelings are obviously shaped by difference but are surely not bound by difference, or so she thought to herself. At some fundamental level we all feel, and feelings – hurt, pain, love, fear – are all aspects of the human experience that bind us together. Troubles happen when we think our pain is different or worse than someone else's, but the reality is that unbearable pain is unbearable pain to the person experiencing it, whatever the cause.

She thought of Carl Rogers' work in encounter groups (Rogers, 1970), and in particular working in areas of conflict, trying to bring people together (Rogers, 1980, 1986, 1987). So often it was about people realising that what-ever their differences, whatever the sections of society they identified with and what terrible things they might inflict on another group of people, the bottom line was that they all hurt and that hurt had a commonality to it. Hurt is hurt. If people could really listen to and hear the hurt that they cause others, and could really connect with their own inner hurt over what they may have done or contributed to, then there is hope of reconciliation. But it has to be rooted in shared feelings, it has to touch the core of a person's being to be authentic, real and potentially contribute to a sustainable change in attitude.

Summary

Fareeda brings a poem written by her son. Carla is deeply moved by it and it leads Fareeda into connecting with powerful emotions. It brings Fareeda and Carla closer and in the process Fareeda breaks through an inner barrier in order to hold Carla. She does not mention this. Fareeda is exhausted by the emotional release and spends the rest of the session sitting quietly with a cup of tea before leaving early.

Points for discussion

- Do you feel that the supervision session fully and appropriately addressed the issues that needed to be raised? Are there issues of race, religion or culture that should have been explored further?
- How did you experience William's supervisory style? Do you feel it was helpful?
- How was Carla communicating unconditional positive regard in counselling session 2?
- Do you feel that Carla was able to be different in counselling session 2 as a result of her supervision session?
- How were you left feeling as you read the poem that Fareeda brought, and how might you have responded had that been given to you by a client?
- How did you respond to Fareeda feeling she might want to establish a strong Islamic identity? Could you empathise with this?
- What are the key characteristics of a counsellor that will enable a client to engage with and release deep pain, and what characteristics might obstruct this?
- Making a client a cup of tea during a session following an intensely emotional experience – consider the appropriateness of this action from the standpoint of person-centred theory.
- Write your own notes for counselling session 2.

CHAPTER 4

Counselling session 3: Wednesday 1st April – spirituality, prayers and an exchange of gifts

The session had begun with Fareeda talking about her reaction to the previous session; how it had calmed her, but not for long, that things had become worse at home with Ali reacting against the suggestion that he might have a drug problem. He had become violent and broken a door. His father had declared that he had had enough, that Ali would have to leave if he couldn't control himself. It led to a huge row and what now amounted to a stand-off.

'I've tried talking to him but he doesn't want to see anyone. Keeps saying he's had enough of shrinks. No one wants to help him and that he feels better smoking cannabis. He's really frightening me. He's spoken a couple of times now about voices telling him it's OK to do what he's doing. I'm really afraid something is going badly wrong. He hasn't been violent any more and things have settled a bit the last couple of days; it was over the weekend when things were really bad. But I don't know what to do. He won't accept there's a problem. What do I do?'

Carla realised that things were serious. 'Fareeda, I'm coming out of counselling here as I think we need to discuss what is happening to Ali and his needs. I'm not qualified to comment in any diagnostic manner, and to be honest I am not sure that diagnoses are necessarily helpful – people can end up labelled and that can be a problem. However, I do know that cannabis can be linked to triggering psychotic episodes, possibly more so the 'skunk' cannabis, though I'm certainly no expert on that and, well, I'm not saying that is happening but I do think you need to let your GP know what is happening, and you do have a right to request a mental health assessment of him.'

Are these grounds for the counsellor to offer direct advice? The counsellor has been informed of a situation that could suggest harm to Ali if the voices he is hearing change. Is this indicative of a psychotic state? It is important not to over-react and perhaps what happens in this narrative is an over-reaction. The counsellor must decide how they would respond, or would they continue to empathise with the client and maybe make a comment at the end of the session? That would be another way of responding. But I include this development within the narrative in order to raise the issue. As mentioned earlier, some will say that mental health diagnoses are not a part of person-centred theory, however, at what point should a counsellor be prepared to offer direct advice where someone in the family is experiencing symptoms that could be associated with psychosis, which, perhaps more importantly, might become a factor in behaviours that could be harmful to the client or others?

'I'm just so worried. I mean, I come back home now as quick as I can, wondering how he will be. It's on my mind all day. I know that at times I'm not really concentrating properly at work. My line manager has noticed and had words about how I seem preoccupied. I said I had family problems – didn't want to say too much. But the thought of getting mental health services involved ... I really don't have much faith that they will help.'

'It's a difficult area, and you're worried, of course you are, and it's distracting you and, yes, from past experience you are not very comfortable with the idea of getting mental health services involved.'

Fareeda was shaking her head. 'I wish he'd talk to someone, someone like you. But he's adamant that he doesn't have a problem and just wants everyone to get off his case.'

'I can appreciate your reluctance. And he could simply be creating in his head the idea of voices telling him to carry on using the cannabis. It could be self-generated to stop him questioning what he is doing.'

'He's not questioning what he is doing, Carla, and I can't seem to get him to question it either. I was shocked when he reacted so at the weekend, he really did lose it. I've seen him react, but this was different. He somehow didn't seem himself. I was concerned he would hurt himself.'

'Hurt himself?'

Fareeda nodded. 'I don't think he was a danger to any of us. Yes, he swore and shouted – but so did Chris. Ali must be in such inner turmoil at the moment and I can't seem to reach him, but I want to, desperately. And when he said about hearing voices telling him to smoke, I really wasn't sure what to do. It only happened yesterday and I thought I'd mention it today. And yes, I need to talk to Dr Martin. And see what he thinks. But he may not know. I mean, maybe I should talk to the drug people as well. They really did seem clued up.'

'Maybe you do need to do both.'

How might we view the phenomenon of hearing voices from a person-centred perspective? A person who has been traumatised to the point of generating dissociated states within their self-structure could well hear voices from parts of themselves prompting certain behaviours. It would be consistent with person-centred theory as it has been developed in recent years in terms of dissociative process (Warner, 2000). Is there something psycho-pathological where voices are heard? What governs this diagnosis? The nature of the messages? The behaviours that follow? Or the simple fact of hearing a voice? It is complicated and perhaps more than a psychological phenomenon in response to traumatic experiencing.

There has also been a long-running debate as to whether cannabis use can trigger psychotic episodes, or does it simply bring them out in people who already carry a previously unrecognised predisposition for such experiences? One might therefore wonder whether certain substances could exacerbate dissociative experiences, leading to more complex and disturbing processes within the psyche of the person.

However, the experiences may not be linked to dissociation, but perhaps to the idea that there are 'parts' within a person's structure of self, 'configurations within self', as proposed by Mearns (Mearns and Thorne, 2000), which emerge from normal development as opposed to dissociative states which tend to develop in response to traumatic experience (Warner, 2000, 2002).

It seems appropriately professional for Carla to address the issue now that it has been raised and for her to help Fareeda decide what course of action to take. It might be debatable as to whether Carla being so directive in her comments is consistent with person-centred working. However, I would argue that this is an occasion when it is appropriate. Without exploring what has occurred further, an opportunity may be lost for Fareeda to explore the likely need to take action. The voices are already urging Ali to act in a way that is potentially causing damage (smoking cannabis) – though in fact the motivating impulse could be to help him avoid or suppress disturbing feelings or thoughts by smoking in order to self-medicate.

For Carla there was always a question of what was going to be helpful for someone like Ali. She had herself encountered clients who heard voices and for her it was a matter of trying to understand what the purpose in the voices was. What were they trying to communicate? What meaning did they have for the client? She would work with them, seeking to hold them as precious parts, equally in need of feeling heard. But she also knew that there was a line over which she would not cross and at which point she would encourage the client to consider psychiatric help. In fact, she had on one occasion negotiated with a client to call her GP and make an appointment to see him, which she did, and as a result the client was referred for a psychiatric assessment. But she based that judgement on the fact that the voices were threatening and the client was feeling unsafe and wanted to protect herself from what was happening.

Carla felt that there were times when clients needed protection for their own well-being, and she knew that perhaps not everyone would agree. Yes, she trusted the process, she trusted the presence of the actualising tendency, and she realised that for her there was a limit, there were phenomena, experiences, behaviours that threatened to put the client or others at risk, and she was not prepared to leave that risk unaddressed. She recognised that there were times when the client's clearly fragile state and communicated lack of safety was an expression of their need for help beyond what was available within the counselling relationship.

Fareeda knew that she did need to contact Dr Martin and the drug team, and she knew she also needed to try and talk to Ali again herself. She felt she needed some more advice on this. She asked Carla what she thought.

'I wish I had the answer, Fareeda, I wish I knew what could be said that would be helpful. I suppose that for me it comes down to what you want to tell him, what you want him to hear.'

'I want him to let me in. I want him to know how much I care, how much I love him, how worried I am, how it's affecting me, but most of all my fear for what is happening to him.' Fareeda was looking down again as she spoke. Ali was her elder son but he was retreating from her. And there was Adam. He was getting caught up in all of this. He seemed to go out more these days, didn't seem to want to be around the house. He'd also been angry at times, and said how he hated the tension in the house, that he couldn't feel comfortable. He had a couple of good friends who lived nearby and he spent a lot of time with them. It seemed to Fareeda that in a way she was at risk of losing him as well. And Chris, well, she thought she still loved him but she wondered why sometimes. He was just so black and white about things, and so self-centred in wanting the kind of life and home that he wanted. But it wasn't going to be that way. They had problems, but he didn't seem prepared or able to face up to that. He just seemed to react all the time.

'And that fear is very present, very real, just what will happen to Ali?' Carla took a deep breath aware of just how far-reaching her words were. What is going to happen to Ali? A minute-to-minute concern for Fareeda. Never knowing, and probably often expecting the worst.

'I pray for him, Carla, I pray for him so much. I pray that he will be protected. I pray that he decides to stop smoking the cannabis and talk to me, or to someone, anyone, it doesn't have to be me, though I hope it will be . . .' Fareeda paused as she recited in Arabic to herself two prayers she had learned many years before, and which she often recited during the day. 'Fallaho khairun hafeza wa howa arhamur rahimeen.' She paused. 'Hasbunallaho wanemalwakeel.'

Carla waited for a moment or two after Fareeda had finished. 'Do they translate into English?'

'Yes, the first says, "Allah is the best guardian and He is the most Merciful." The second says that, "God sufficeth for us and he is the best Protector." '

Carla was moved by the words and said so. 'Simple yet affirming, very powerful and moving; His mercy and His protection.'

'The best and only kind.'

'Thank you. Thank you for sharing these words. The sounds they make seem poetic and lyrical.'

'They are important to me. As is my belief that Allah is good. There is a reason for all of this. I must apply myself, perhaps I should be praying more.' She paused. 'There is another prayer that I use daily, called the "Dua-E-Jameelah". It helps me to focus on God's qualities. It does not fully translate into English, at least, not the version that I have, but it does help me to remember that God is good, and I hold on to this.'

Carla wanted to hear the prayer, but also wanted to respect Fareeda in her choice not to tell her if that is what she wished. Carla was unsure whether there was any stipulation as to when particular prayers might be used, or whether the words could be recited other than during the act of prayer. 'It sounds very important to you, Fareeda. And I don't know the circumstances in which you would use this prayer, but I would appreciate having a copy in English if that is possible.'

'Really?'

Carla nodded. 'I don't know enough about Islamic prayers and it would be good for me to learn more. It would also help me, I think, to appreciate more how important these prayers are to you.' Carla paused before continuing. 'I have to be honest, I don't pray much, I never have, but I am touched by the way that you are speaking and I appreciate how important it is, how much a part of your life.'

'I'll bring you in a copy . . .' She paused herself and picked up her bag. 'You can have my copy. I have others at home.' She found what she was looking for, a folded sheet of paper with a photocopy of the prayer she had mentioned just previously. 'Here.' She handed it to Carla.

'Are you sure?'

'Yes, of course I am.'

Carla took it. She was genuinely grateful. 'Thank you. I really appreciate this.'

'And I appreciate your wanting a copy. I don't think anyone has ever asked me for a copy of an Islamic prayer, well, not someone who is outside of the Islamic faith.'

What makes it therapeutically significant is that Carla's interest and request is coming from a genuine interest. She is touched by what Fareeda is saying and how she is saying it. She is describing something extremely precious to her and it is important that when this happens in sessions – whatever the subject – that it is handled sensitively and with, I think, a sense of reverence and respect. This exchange of a prayer is representing an exchange of gifts. Carla receives the prayer, Fareeda receives the gift of being heard and of something precious to her being respected. So much of the healing power of the therapeutic relationship, it seems to me, is linked to a notion of exchanging gifts.

'Maybe they need to be more widely available.' Carla was reading it. 'There's nothing here that could offend anyone, it's an acknowledgement of the qualities of God.'

'Yes. And there is only one God, we, of course, call him Allah.'

Carla nodded. That, she thought, was such a fundamental truth that seemed to get lost in all the divisions in the world based on religious belief.

Fareeda was continuing, 'And I like to repeat this prayer at least once a day, and take time to dwell on each of the qualities, and try to imagine myself having those qualities.'

'Thank you, Fareeda, I really, really appreciate this.' Carla carefully placed it on the table beside her. 'I can see something of why it is so important. Something, as you say, to hold on to. Focusing on these qualities.'

'It helps to bring me closer to Allah. It reminds me that He is all of these qualities and, well, strengthens my awareness that all is His creation and my place in life is to be clear as to what His will is for me.'

'Being clear so that you can serve His will, is that what you mean?'

'Yes. Yes, very much so.' Talking like this affected Fareeda. It gave her strength. It reinforced for her that she had to act to help her son. She knew that anyway, but the last few minutes had not so much deepened as reconnected her with what she knew was right and her duty.

Carla nodded, and smiled. She felt huge compassion for Fareeda, and for the role that her faith had in defining her purpose in life. To serve God, to serve Allah. Whilst this was not her belief or view of life, she felt a respect for Fareeda.

'I really do experience great respect for you and for the place your faith has in your life.' Carla was genuine in her words. There was a stillness present in the room.

Fareeda nodded. 'It is important to me. I do not consider myself to be a devout Muslim, but I do read the Koran and say prayers, and I do try to be modest and improve myself for the greater Glory of Allah. My parents were much stricter than I am, and my sons, well, they are not really that drawn to religion, but maybe they'll both change. It saddens me that they are not, but I want them to have the freedom to choose.'

'That sounds really important to you as well.'

'It is. I do try, and I'm sure that, well, there is a purpose to everything I'm having to struggle with, but it's hard to see. Maybe I'm not meant to know, just have to keep trying to do the best I can. I just hope that things change for Ali. And, well, what we said earlier, yes, I do need to talk to Dr Martin and to the drug team. Otherwise I'm sure things can only get worse and I don't want that.' Fareeda suddenly looked so small as she sat there, facing, as far as Carla could sense, such a tremendous challenge. And yet there was something about her. She was clearly not going to give in. It seemed that she had a strong faith which helped her.

'Yes, and I want to acknowledge what I experience as a lot of strength in you, and yet it must feel so overwhelming as well.'

> Carla responds in a way that acknowledges her sense of Fareeda's strength and her own experience of seeing Fareeda as being quite small, facing so much. It is therefore a response partly empathic to Fareeda and partly a congruent communication of Carla's own inner sense.

Fareeda found it hard to own it as being her strength. God's, maybe, but not her's. She didn't feel very strong and at times felt positively weak. But she wasn't going to give up on Ali. He needed help and she was going to make sure he got it. 'I don't think I have much strength, not really. It's not my strength. I pray and, well, I'm sure I am helped. That's what I believe. It is written in the Koran that: "On no soul doth God, Place a burden greater, Than it can bear." ' (Ali, 1938, p. 116)

Although Carla did not have this kind of faith she was very much struck by the power of what Fareeda was saying. She couldn't imagine herself what it must be like to have faith in a God, but she could see how it was helping her client to cope. 'It must be such an important part of, well, I'm not sure what to say, everything, I guess.'

Fareeda nodded. 'It is. And Islam is such a peaceful and gentle religion at heart, it really is. Such beautiful texts and prayers. It is about codes of conduct, about how we should behave towards each other to the greater Glory of Allah's creation. But I see people using Islam as a basis for committing atrocities and it's just not how it should be.' She sighed. 'It saddens me so much. I'm sure people use religion for personal gain and power, to further their own ideas and beliefs. But I guess that can be said of most religions. The true, spiritual heart of the teachings gets lost somehow.' She paused again to take another deep breath. 'Why can't we all live together in peace? Why do we have to have a world where there is such inequality, where difference is feared and governments act in ways that simply inflame hatreds that seem to go back over the generations. When will we learn to forgive and start again?' Fareeda spoke with such a heartfelt yearning. She was so tired of the way Islam was portrayed and misused. It wasn't the religion she knew. 'There is a book, called *The Sayings of Muhammed*. It is a beautiful book of sayings and somehow these are not heard, but they should be. Some in particular stay with me: "Muhammed was asked to curse the infidels, and He answered: 'I was not sent to curse the infidels but to have mercy on mankind' " (Hadith, p. 325)*. And another, "The person who has one atom of pride in his heart will not enter Paradise" (Hadith, p. 37).'

'That seems a long way from what we see of Islam on our televisions and in the newspapers, and, of course, what we see happening in places where there is conflict.'

'Yes, and it does make me sad. I wish these sayings could be publicised more. I do not know the true history of them, but they are beautiful and give important values to live by. If just one tabloid newspaper printed them, well, maybe it might shame some people into thinking differently. There is one other piece,

---

*Quotations from the *Hadith* or 'Table Talk of Muhammed' are from Joseph Gaer (1958) Dodd, Mead & Co., New York, which I have taken from *Everyone is Right* by Roland Peterson (1986) De Vorss & Co., California, in which the author comments that these were taken from Allama Sir Abdulla Al-Manum Al-Suhrowardy *The Sayings of Muhammed*, and published in *The Wisdom of the East* series in London. The numbers correspond to the numbers in *The Sayings of Muhammed*.

more than any other, that stands out for me. Funny, really, given my own belief in prayer. However, it really does put everything in perspective: "Shall I tell you what are better acts than fasting, charity and prayers? Making peace between enemies are such acts; for enmity and malice tear up the heavenly rewards by the roots" (Hadith, p. 340). Making peace, that's what matters, putting hatred and malice aside. That's the true essence of Islam as far as I am concerned. The people who kill believing they will enter paradise, in truth they "tear up the heavenly rewards by the roots". Quite what will happen to them when they die with such malice and hate in their hearts; Islam also talks about intent and action. It seems that people are made to believe that the intent to "kill infidels" as in some way serving the will of Allah justifies murderous action.' She shook her head. 'It is hard sometimes to have a faith that is so distorted by others. I want to be proud of my faith, and I am, but these people, well . . .' She shook her head. 'It makes me sad, and it makes me angry as well. Perhaps I should feel compassion. I guess that is what Allah would want of me.' She sighed.

Carla had listened intently to what Fareeda had been saying. She had spoken from the heart, her words conveyed a view of Islam that Carla appreciated hearing. 'I'm really grateful to you for sharing these sayings. They are very moving and inspiring. And I so hear your sadness, and anger, at the way your faith is used by others who seem bent only on destruction.'

For Fareeda it felt so good to talk like this. She hadn't really spoken in this way for, well, she couldn't remember when. Though it was increasing her sadness and anger it was also helping her to feel that connection, that sense or touch of something deeper within herself. The stillness remained, and it felt strong and pure and clear, like still water. The image of a lake, the water still and clear, yet what potential it had for giving life, and what power it held were it to be released. She thought of Allah as that vast lake, his power, his waters of life, waiting to be powerfully released. 'Why can't we live together in peace?'

Carla took a deep breath, it was her turn to sigh. 'Yes, why can't we live together in peace?' She did not voice it as a question to Fareeda, but more to the world, and to herself. 'Was it not Ghandi who said that we must become the change we wish to see in the world, or something like that. To see peace we must become peaceful, I guess, we must be and encourage the attitudes that we would want to see governing human hearts and minds.' Carla was aware that she wasn't really being a therapist, at least not in the normal sense, and yet somehow she did feel engaged with Fareeda in a therapeutic process. She was listening to what Fareeda was saying, feeling warm acceptance towards her and seeking to be in touch with her own experience in response to what Fareeda was saying.

Carla has directed Fareeda back to her personal focus by her comment. She has stepped out of a therapy role in, perhaps, a traditional sense, and yet she has engaged with Fareeda over matters of importance. What prompted Carla to mention Ghandi's words, only she can know. Perhaps in the relational flow the time was right for the focus to move back and it happened to be Carla that was the one voicing this move. Perhaps there can be times in the therapeutic process when it is quite acceptable to introduce an idea or a response that has a directive impact. Or is this an attempt to justify a response that was, whilst well intentioned within the dialogue, clearly directive?

It is perhaps worth remembering Rogers' comment concerning behaviours and actions of the therapist when there is a sense of deep, inner connection: 'When I am at my best, as a group facilitator or as a therapist, I discover another characteristic. I find that when I am closest to my inner, intuitive self, when I am somehow in touch with the unknown in me, when perhaps I am in a slightly altered state of consciousness, then whatever I do seems to be full of healing. Then, simply my *presence* is releasing and helpful to the other. There is nothing I can do to force this experience, but when I can relax and be close to the transcendent core of me, then I may behave in strange and impulsive ways in the relationship, ways which I cannot justify rationally, which have nothing to do with my thought processes. But these strange behaviours turn out to be *right*, in some odd way: it seems that my inner spirit has reached out and touched the inner spirit of the other. Our relationship transcends itself and becomes a part of something larger. Profound growth and healing and energy are present.' (Rogers, 1980, p. 129)

It can seem confusing, when to speak and when not to. When to trust that inner urge and when to dismiss it as irrelevant and a distraction. Perhaps the litmus test lies in the therapist's sense of depth and connectedness in the moment of experiencing an urge to speak.

We might conclude that there can be occasions within the therapeutic process when the connection and focus have a certain transcending quality and perhaps, in those moments, a momentary new order of relationship emerges. An urge to say something may arise that is of an order beyond the usual urge to speak, that may be coloured by personal issues and values. Some would say that, if this process occurs, then perhaps it is a soul or higher self prompting what is said, a part of human nature that transcends the separateness of everyday body-bound experience. Or, if we take the view that God exists and does 'speak' to us occasionally, why should this voice not be heard in the therapy room?

Fareeda felt her focus switch to the more immediate and personal. 'And sometimes I don't feel very peaceful, and, well, I can't be, not really. I need to be angry sometimes, or at least people make me angry. I get angry with Chris, and I've been angry with people who haven't helped Ali but who have, I felt, somewhat condescendingly just put his mood down to "being a teenager".' She shook her head. 'I don't feel very peaceful sometimes, I want to make war, make people listen. And I'm probably going to have to do this now to make sure Ali gets help. It never ends, not when you're seen as different, when you're a different colour and speak with a different accent.'
'No chance of peace when you need to make war to get the help Ali needs. An ongoing struggle because your skin is a different colour and you have a different

accent.' Carla could feel herself involuntarily shaking her head slightly. She stopped herself from speaking just as the words 'when are we going to learn?' were about to pass her lips. She sat, feeling her own sense of despair at humanity's seeming inability to respect and honour difference rather than fear it and use it as a reason to inflict suffering on others.

Empathy is a challenge when a client is exploring a theme that is triggering a process within the counsellor. There may be times when this will need to be made visible – perhaps particularly if it becomes a block to accurate empathy. Otherwise, it should be noted but not dwelt on, enabling the counsellor to remain focused on, and therapeutically connected to, the client.

The session continued with Fareeda exploring further her own sense of despair, and towards the end of the session she brought the focus back to her son. 'I guess the world is like Ali, trying to avoid pain and yet ending up causing more pain, and suffering, and damage. I'll make some calls when I get back home. God willing, he's going to get the help he needs.'

The session drew to a close. It was after Fareeda had left that Carla again picked up the prayer that she had left. She read it slowly and thoughtfully, she didn't understand all the words, but those that she did certainly seemed to her to be expressive of qualities that she would associate with God – if she believed in God. She read through the qualities listed.

O Virtues! O Allah O Near! O Allah O Wonderful! O Allah O Acceptor! O Allah O Benevolent! O Allah O Virtuous! O Allah O Obliging! O Allah O Dyyan! O Allah O Reason! O Allah O Mighty! O Allah O Helper! O Allah O Obliger! O Allah O The Greatest! O Allah O Benevolent! O Allah O Merciful! O Allah O Clement! O Allah O Knower ! O Allah O Bountiful! O Allah O Great! O Allah O Majeed! O Allah O Wise! O Allah O Powerful! O Allah O Forgiver! O Allah O Forgiver of sins! O Allah O Creator! O Allah O Exalting! O Allah O Appreciator of Thankfuls! O Allah O Knower! O Allah O Seer! O Allah O Hearer! O Allah O The First! O Allah O The Last! O Allah O Appearance! O Allah O Essence! O Allah O Pious! O Allah O Protector! O Allah O Watcher! O Allah O Dear! O Allah O Great! O Allah O Creating! O Allah O Possessor! O Allah O Artist! O Allah O Tremendous! O Allah O Living! O Allah O Immortal! O Allah O Limiter! O Allah O Expander! O Allah O Abasing! O Allah O Energizing! O Allah O Existing! O Allah O Giver! O Allah O Eliminator! O Allah O Sublimer! O Allah O Guardian! O Allah O Helper! O Allah O Great! O Allah O Merciful! O Allah O Shower of the way! O Allah O Sober! O Allah O Opener! O Allah.

She was struck by the impact it had on her. She felt quite calm, and somehow humbled and yet uplifted. It was powerful. She thoughtfully placed it back down on the table.

Summary

Fareeda talks about her son hearing voices and Carla encourages her to consider speaking to someone about it. Fareeda agrees. She also mentioned how difficult it has been in the past getting help for Ali, how she has had to struggle, and how she feels much of the difficulty was linked to her different skin colour and accent, making it feel as if she was not deserving of services. She then talks about Islam and shares some prayers and sayings that have particular meaning to her. A deeper, spiritual focus emerges. Carla is moved by what Fareeda says and after the session reads a prayer that she has left for her, having only had time to glance over it during the actual counselling session.

Counselling session 4: Wednesday 8th April – the client's son has a 'psychotic' episode and is in hospital

The session had begun and Fareeda had been describing her week. Ali's mental state had deteriorated to the point that Fareeda had called her GP and asked him to visit. He came and realised straight away that something was seriously wrong. Yes, Ali had been smoking and was somewhat 'out of it', but he had been talking to himself and acting rather bizarrely around the house. He had seemed to get very nervous whenever he was outside of his room, looking around anxiously, muttering to himself. The doctor had got him admitted into the local psychiatric unit after Ali had reluctantly accepted this.

Fareeda went back over the events leading up to Dr Martin arriving. 'It was awful, I didn't know what to do. He was just, I don't know, it's hard to describe, he moved in an odd sort of way, and his eyes, I mean, he just looked sort of blank and staring at the same time, agitated, bewildered, I can't really describe it. It was like he was there but not there. But he kept looking around, he wouldn't settle. I tried to calm him down but he just wouldn't, couldn't.' Fareeda was back reliving the experience, she could see him clearly and felt her own anxiety. He had seemed somehow 'other-worldly'.

Fareeda continued talking. 'I prayed, I was saying my prayers all the time, hoping that he would settle down again. It seemed an age before Dr Martin arrived. It was like, oh it's too awful to say, but, well, it seemed like he was possessed, just not Ali. It was like it was my son but it wasn't.' At this Fareeda felt the tears in her eyes. She hadn't really talked much about it, not like this anyway. Chris hadn't really listened in the same way that Carla was, and her sister was away, visiting family back in Mauritius. Carla didn't say much – she didn't need to – but to Fareeda she seemed to be so attentive, she felt her presence so clearly, watching, listening, being there. 'I really thought he was going mad. He wanted to go back into his room, and I persuaded him to let me come in with him, though he didn't want me to. Kept saying it was the only place he could be safe, that he could get away from "them". I didn't know what he meant. He wouldn't say, just kept acting strangely.'

Carla could see how distraught Fareeda was just in recounting what had happened, how it must have affected her at the time she could only imagine. Her heart went out to her – her son being the way she was describing him. It sounded as though he was having a psychotic episode. She didn't try to be clever though with an explanation, she nodded and empathised with what had been said. 'So he had to be in the bedroom to feel safe, to get away from them, and it really felt like he was going mad?'

Fareeda nodded. It really had. He'd had weird attacks in the past, but nothing on the scale of what had occurred this time. 'I kept trying to calm him down. There wasn't anyone else around. Adam was out and Chris hadn't got home from work. I actually called Chris as well, he seemed more irritated than concerned. I hung up on him, I had to stay with Ali until the doctor arrived, he just didn't seem safe.'

'Must have felt like a long wait, on your own, and not getting much support from Chris.'

'Bastard. I think I've had enough of him.' Fareeda's face was suddenly very hard and her jaw was set firm. 'But that's something else.' She paused, thinking about her marriage. Yes, it had been good to begin with but over the years, and particularly with the problems that Ali had had, they had drifted apart. She seemed to have to cope with him on her own, and she believed strongly in the family, in working at things, but she knew that maybe it was only a matter of time. But she couldn't see how she could leave and be able to look after Ali. She felt trapped. Her heart sank. The expression on her face changed and Carla noticed this.

'You look suddenly very sad.'

'Thinking about my marriage, what it's become and just, oh I don't know, trying to cope with it all.' She took a deep breath and sighed. 'Something else to sort out, add it to the list.' She smiled weakly.

Carla nodded, aware that Fareeda had shifted the focus of what she was saying. She stayed with where Fareeda was in her self now.

Person-centred therapy requires the counsellor to remain in contact with the client as they move around within themselves. By being allowed to talk about the events with Ali, Fareeda has connected with other thoughts and feelings, and these must be warmly accepted and the counsellor needs to communicate that she has heard what has been said.

'Sounds like it's a long list, Fareeda, on top of everything else is your marriage which brings you a lot of sadness.'

'Only some of it. Chris, mainly. He's just so unhelpful and, well, he and Ali, I've said before, I just feel in the middle so much. It's horrible.'

'Horrible being in the middle.'

For Fareeda it was a place where she simply felt she couldn't win. She couldn't agree with Chris's attitude and in effect abandon Ali, and she found it so hard to cope with Chris's attitude when she gave her time to her son. Her son, yes, that's how it is, her son. For some reason this idea struck her forcibly. She hadn't quite thought of it like that before, at least, not so powerfully. Another deep breath.

'You look very much lost in thought.'

Fareeda nodded. 'I just realised, and it sounds an awful thing to say, but, well, it feels like Ali's no longer our son, it feels like he's only mine. I mean, I'm sure that deep down it's not like that, but it is how it feels. I was just thinking and it struck me that really Ali's my son, not our son. That also saddens me as well. Ali needs his father. But Chris can't seem to, or doesn't want to, well, even try and understand. So, you see, I'm all Ali's got. I have to keep going, keep being there for him. I have to.' It seemed to Fareeda that although her son was such a challenge, she knew she loved him and she really wanted to be there for him. And she knew she would always be there for him, but always suddenly felt like an awfully long time.

Carla nodded, 'You have to keep going, no one else, it's all down to you, that's how it feels?'

Fareeda nodded again. Her heart felt heavy as she sat staring down at the floor. She hadn't been feeling like this when she had arrived. And whilst she knew she had her down moments, somehow it seemed particularly heavy just at the moment. The words from Ali's poem came into her mind, 'nowhere left to run'. She felt like she had nowhere left to run.

'You know, there are times when I'd like to just hide in my room, and shut the world out. I can really sympathise with Ali in a way, he must so want to get away from what he feels. Anyway, he's stable again now. They plan to let him back home at the end of the week and they're referring him to the drug team as well. They've already sent someone in to see him. So I just pray that it works. I don't know if I could go through all of this again.'

'Bit like Ali, get away, hide away. He uses cannabis to get away . . .'

'Yes, and I, well, I have nothing, well, apart from work. But that's not the answer, is it? And I just think about Ali, worry about him, I never get away. You don't, do you, that's part of being a mother?'

'So you feel you have nothing to help you really get away.' Carla wondered about Fareeda's other son. She was very conscious, suddenly, of how little she spoke of him. But this was not what Fareeda was speaking about so she let it go, but not without noting a wonder in her self what their relationship must be like.

Fareeda nodded. 'No. But, well, God willing, things will work out for him, for us. I have to believe that, I really have to.' She paused before continuing. 'I just hope that things settle down this time, but, well, Ali was so bad. He was saying some really crazy things by the time Dr Martin arrived, talking about people spying on him, that people were outside listening through the walls, that his room was the only safe place to be, and that smoking the cannabis really put up a smoke screen, filled him full of smoke so they couldn't see him or read his mind.' Fareeda shook her head.

Carla could appreciate the craziness of a psychotic episode, and she also appreciated that Ali's inner world needed to be understood, that he maybe needed someone to help him feel less alone in that frightening, paranoid place inside himself. She didn't think there was a good enough appreciation and understanding that psychotic episodes may seem like some kind of madness from the outside, but the form they took was likely to have meaning for the client. Was it ever explored? Why should Ali feel the way he did? Why did he feel spied on? Why did he feel a need to hide behind a smoke screen? What was he hiding from? He would need some sensitive therapeutic work at some point, but it seemed to her that so often this wasn't available, almost as if the actual psychotic experience was out of bounds to explore – perhaps a fear that talking about it could trigger it again. But it had to be understood. Psychotic episodes had meaning for clients, they took the form they did for a reason, or so she believed.

How does a person-centred counsellor work with a client who is experiencing a psychotic episode? There is the view that psychiatric diagnosis is not a component of the person-centred model, nevertheless the question remains regarding how to work with a client who is experiencing what are termed 'psychotic symptoms'. The key question is whether there is sufficient 'psychological contact'? The client may be so engaged in his or her own inner worlds of experience and may be so cut off from the outer world in which the therapist has their focus, that the degree of psychological contact, indeed if there is any at all, becomes a topic of debate.

The development of what is termed 'pre-therapy' (Prouty, 2002; Prouty *et al.*, 2002) has provided a major theoretical development to the practice of working with clients for whom the nature, depth or even existence of psychological contact is under question. Within Rogers' system, psychological contact is the first necessary and sufficient condition for constructive personality change (Rogers, 1957). Prouty defines pre-therapy in the following terms, as 'the development of restoration of the functions necessary for a therapeutic relationship and experiencing. Pre-therapy, described in general terms, develops the necessary psychological capacities for psychotherapy. It assists those clients who are impaired in the psychological functions for treatment to occur' (Prouty, 2002, p. 55).

Prouty describes a series of contact functions which he indicates as representing an expansion of Perls' concept of 'contact and ego function'; these contact functions being 'conceived as awareness functions and described as reality, affective and communicative contact', and it is 'the development or restoration of the contact functions' that is 'the necessary pre-condition for psychotherapy'. It is the development or restoration of the contact functions that is the theoretical goal of pre-therapy (Prouty, 2002, p. 58), and at the core of this process lies the notion of 'contact reflections'. These have the 'theoretical function of developing psychological contact between therapist and client when the client is incapable of reality, affective or communicative contact. They are applied when there is not sufficient contact to implement psychotherapy' (Prouty, 2002, pp. 55–6). There are five 'contact reflections' (Karon and Vanderbos, 1981): 'situational reflections, facial reflections, word-for-word reflections, body reflections and reiterative reflections.'

'So he hid in the smoke, in the safety of his room. In a way that makes sense if you believe there are people he needs to hide from.'
'I know. And as I say, I can appreciate that there are times I want to hide away, well, maybe not hide, more just get away. But he talked of hiding.' She remembered past experiences with Ali. 'But of course he has tried to get away as well. The trip to Wales, to the mountains, and other times he's just up and gone. There is something about getting away as well as hiding away. What's he getting away from, Carla?' She shook her head, feeling desperate in her wanting to know what was driving her son to behave as he did.
'I guess that's what needs to be understood.'
'Well, I hope he sees someone who approaches it like this, I really do. I don't want him on some medication to drug him up that doesn't really address the issue. I want my son back. I want him to find release from his nightmare, Carla, am I asking too much?'
Carla shook her head.
'That's what I pray for, to have my son back, for him to be free of the nightmare, free of the thoughts and feelings, from whatever it is that drives him. She shook her head again. ' "Nowhere left to run"; those words make me go cold. Whatever was he thinking when he wrote those words, well, not just that, what was he feeling, how was he feeling? How was he feeling, Carla?' Fareeda looked searchingly into Carla's eyes. Carla held Fareeda's silent gaze, the gaze of a mother desperately reaching out, wanting answers where there didn't seem to be any, wanting to understand, wanting reassurance that she was a good mother, wanting to feel supported, wanting to feel something, anything, other than the pressure and the anxiety, the uncertainty and confusion that filled her waking life – and no doubt her sleep as well.
Carla could sense that Fareeda was feeling so much inside, but she wasn't communicating anything specifically. Carla wasn't in a place in herself to think about how to respond; she felt in contact with Fareeda and trusted herself to respond freely and openly as felt right, trusting that the psychological contact would direct her.

Can the counsellor truly trust her instinct, or should it be called intuition, when strong psychological contact is present in the therapeutic relationship? Some might argue that this contact goes beyond two people sitting in separate bodies in a room; the counsellor experiencing their own inner reactions to what the client is experiencing and communicating. Could the contact be more tangible, albeit invisible? Could there be some real connection established at some subtle, energetic level? Could the potent directing force of the actualising tendency of the client somehow connect with the psyche of the counsellor in some mysterious way that draws out of the therapist the response that the client's actualising tendency needs to feed off? Or is this fantasy? Are there mechanisms of subtle contact that transcend the five senses? If so, then it seems that they need to be embraced and acknowledged as significant factors within the therapeutic relationship.

Carla heard herself speak. 'I don't know, Fareeda, I sense your desperate need to know, but I don't have an answer to that question. Only Ali can answer that.'

Fareeda nodded. Yes, she desperately needed to know, perhaps more than ever now after what had happened. She needed to understand what was driving the way he thought and felt, and acted. 'Yes. You're right. I do know that, and in a way I don't want someone else telling me. At one level I do, but deep down it's Ali, I need to know from him, I need him to tell me.' The tears welled up in her eyes and she reached for a tissue.

Carla felt the emotion of the moment too. She felt such heart-rending compassion for Fareeda, desperately wanting to communicate with her son, to understand from him what he was going through, to find ways, as his mother, to be with him, to help him through. 'I really feel for you, Fareeda, I wish I had the magic therapeutic wand to make sense of everything and make it all better, but I haven't, and it's probably a daft thing for me to have said anyway.'

'No, somehow I know that if you could wave that magic wand, you would. I know it doesn't exist but, well, I also hope that it does as well, that someone, some-where, will have the answer.' Another deep breath and sigh. Fareeda felt stiff. She'd been sitting not moving for a long while. She shifted her weight in the chair and stretched her back, moving her head slightly from side to side. 'Oh, that's better. I get set if I sit for too long.' She paused. 'No, no magic wand, but I do hope that he gets to see someone, someone really sensitive who can help him explore, make sense of what's going on for him. He's only young. If it can be resolved now, well, maybe he'll have the chance of a much better life in the future. I don't want him drugged up on some awful medicine for the rest of his life, it's not the answer, I know it isn't. He's got to talk to someone.'

'You sound really clear on this, on his need to talk, and to be heard by someone sensitive and responsive to him so he can explore and understand . . .'

'I hope so. I really do. Do you think that'll happen?'

In all honesty, Carla was not sure. 'Like you, I hope so. It's going to be a sensi-tive time for him at the moment; he'll be off the cannabis.' Why am I saying this, Carla thought to herself? I'm not empathising but trying to reassure or give Fareeda a lecture on the effects of stopping using cannabis. And besides, she'd heard that clients could get hold of street drugs sometimes even on so-called secure wards. She pulled herself back into Fareeda's world. 'So, like you, I hope so.'

'There's . . . , I don't know, some kind of meeting at the psychiatric unit tomorrow. I'm going to it, Chris isn't.' She tightened her jaw as she mentioned Chris's name. 'Sort of planning meeting for Ali's discharge. Got a letter about it, seems like someone from the drug team will be there.'

Carla knew what Fareeda meant and she also know how difficult the meetings could be for clients – and family – particularly if a lot of professionals were involved, and she had seen it happen that it could be so prescriptive and quite damaging. She hoped that this would not be Fareeda's experience.

'So you are going, must leave you with thoughts and feelings, I guess?'

Fareeda nodded. 'I have things I need to say, and I guess one thing is about what I think Ali needs. I just hope they listen to me.'

'You want to be heard, Fareeda, and I guess you want to be sure that you say exactly what you want to say?'

Fareeda nodded, aware of feeling concerned that she might not be able to put it how she wanted to, or not feel she was taken seriously. She felt that her ethnic difference might make it more difficult. She'd met the consultant. He'd seemed very able but somehow a bit remote, rather too matter of fact. She hadn't really felt heard by him. It left her feeling anxious about it.

The session continued with a discussion as to how Fareeda could be sure she said what she wanted to say. She decided she would write what she wanted to say, and take a copy to leave for the file. She wanted it in writing, and she was going to copy it to her GP as well. She worked out what she would say and scribbled a few sentences before the end of the session.

She felt good as she left, felt she had something she could do. She wasn't looking forward to the meeting the next day but she knew it was an opportunity, her opportunity to try and ensure that Ali got what she felt he needed, though she knew she would have to make her presence felt for this to have a chance of happening.

Carla felt concern. She knew how difficult these kinds of discharge meeting could be. For anyone faced with a group of professionals with their own ideas as to what was best in the way of treatment, it could seem daunting. For someone with a mental health problem, and for someone from an ethnic minority, it could be even more of a problem. Of course, the idea was to get everyone around the table and formulate a treatment response that would be most effective following discharge. But often the meetings could take on a kind of purely administrative nature, the decisions having already been made and the meeting being to inform the patients and any relative who was present what would be done, and ensuring the necessary paperwork was completed. Was she being a bit too critical? Perhaps. She knew that it wasn't always like this, but she knew that it could be. She was glad Fareeda was going to write a statement. And she was glad that she would be there for Ali as well.

Summary

Ali has been admitted into a psychiatric unit after Fareeda called the doctor. He was acting very strangely. Fareeda describes her husband's response and is sad at the state of her marriage. She talks of praying to have her son back. She has been invited to a meeting at the psychiatric unit. Her husband has refused to attend. Fareeda realises how important it is for her to say what she wants to have heard at the meeting and she discusses with Carla how best to do this.

Points for discussion

- If you had a client telling you that they heard voices, would you feel competent to work with them? At what point might you consider the need for other, specialist interventions?
- Do you feel that Carla was offering a therapeutic response to Fareeda when she was talking about Islam?
- What is your reaction to the spiritual focus in counselling session 3, and the ideas concerning a transcendent core?
- Are there factors that might make it difficult for you to genuinely empathise with Fareeda in counselling session 3? And if so, what would you do about it?
- From a person-centred theoretical perspective, how would you explain the process of what might be termed a 'psychotic episode'?
- Discuss the role of pre-therapy and consider examples from your own work where this might prove helpful, and why.
- How do you respond to the notion that there might be subtle mechanisms of communication beyond the five senses? What are your reasons for your answer?
- If you were Fareeda, writing a statement to present to a discharge meeting for Ali, what would you write, what would you want the professionals to hear and understand?
- Write your own notes for these sessions.

CHAPTER 5

Supervision session 2: Friday 10th April – mental health and person-centred working explored

'So, Fareeda's son had to be hospitalised. I'm wondering about your reaction to that.'

Carla nodded and spoke her thoughts. 'It sounded reasonable. Clearly, things had taken a turn for the worse. I felt for Fareeda, having to cope with what happened on her own, and I hope that things went well at the discharge meeting that she was going to attend. So how do I react? Well, I am aware of feeling very concerned whether being hospitalised and being given powerful medication can have an effect that blocks the client's internal psychological process. I also appreciate that for some people there is simply a need for them to be in a place of safety from where a plan of action can be formulated. Clearly, Ali was losing it. How much was cannabis induced, how much was his own thought processes running to extreme, I don't know. But there's no doubt that Ali does experience some degree of internal pain – I'm not sure what else to call it – psychological or emotional distress?'

'I guess that for me it is about checking whether your reaction to whatever treatment Ali might receive will cloud the clarity of your empathy for whatever Fareeda might be experiencing, when you next see her.'

'Yes, and because I know that I believe, passionately, that he could benefit from some kind of therapy – maybe quite intense – to help him process whatever is happening for him, I may find it difficult to be unbiased in the next and proceeding sessions.'

William nodded, pleased that Carla could recognise this, and he asked her to clarify what she meant by her use of the word 'unbiased'.

'I might carry a negative attitude towards what Ali is offered if it isn't what I believe he should receive. And that might affect my ability to really hear Fareeda. I'm not sure. I can see how easily, if he is not offered, say, some proper therapeutic counselling – and not simply medication to control the symptoms, or keyworking sessions to deal only with controlling his thinking, and/or his cannabis use, at a very cognitive and behavioural level – well, the emotional content, the deeper, internal difficulties may get missed and any, if you like, surface changes may not get underpinned by genuine personal growth and change.'

'So your concern is about whether her son will get the kind of therapy that will go deeper into the meaning of the psychotic episode.'

'And hearing you use that label or diagnosis, I feel a reaction.' Carla didn't like these kinds of label, they always seemed to carry a social stigma. She recognised that was as much about societal fear as anything else, but nevertheless, she knew how easy it was for people to equate psychosis with madness, when for some people it was simply that they experienced themselves differently. That difference may involve taking thought and behavioural processes to extremes, but she felt that somehow there was always scope for understanding, for helping people to explore themselves and, yes, there would be times when there was a genuine chemical imbalance within the person and some form of chemical treatment was required to re-balance the system. She appreciated that and did not have any problems with it, so long as the medication used could strategically impact on the chemical need rather than bring with it a range of side-effects that might contribute to other areas of problematic experience for the client. She also accepted that medication could stabilise someone where this was the case in order to enable them to better engage in therapy. However, she was distrustful of deciding, too soon, that clients were incapable of engaging with someone and medication being used as a first rather than a last resort.

'What kind of reaction?'

Carla described the thoughts that she had and then continued. 'I guess the thing for me is that it is so easy for clients to be blamed for not being co-operative, when in fact it is what they are being offered, and how they are being offered it, that is contributing to them being that way.'

William nodded. 'So, from a person-centred perspective, how would you describe your position?' He felt it would be helpful for Carla to process her reaction, her thoughts and concerns in the light of person-centred theory.

'Well, first of all, there is the fact that someone else is perhaps taking a position of authority.'

'So that authority has implications?'

'Well, once someone has been given a diagnosis then the expert on what that diagnosis means can take over. And, yes, that can be highly appropriate where there is great vulnerability and mental disturbance, but where there is uncertainty over the value or accuracy of the diagnosis, well, then there becomes the risk that the client's meaning and experience – the uniqueness of what has happened to him, or her – can get lost in the generally assumed meaning and nature of that particular diagnosis.'

'So, the specificity of the client's experience gets lost in a general view of what a particular diagnosis means?'

'Yes, and I am concerned that if someone cannot relate effectively to Ali, then the specificity of his experience will not be perhaps as fully communicated and

heard as it might be, and so the general understanding of treatment responses to the diagnosis will be applied without them being informed by the specificity of Ali's experience. Does that make sense, or am I making this sound unclear?'
'No, it sounds clear to me. You are concerned that if there isn't accurate communication between Ali and whoever is assigned to treat him, then he will receive treatment based on general understanding rather than what is specific to his needs, his experiences.'
'And for me it is about the vulnerability of clients with mental health problems who may need a lot of time in order to feel able to communicate the specifics of their experience, who are naturally defensive because, let's say, the underlying cause of their difficulties is some kind of trauma. He may not feel able to disclose an event or series of events for a whole host of reasons, and part of this could be some degree of mental health impairment. I know how clients can need time, and psychiatric units can be intense places, with disturbances. You can have a lot of disturbed people together and I know how people in those settings who are sensitive, who have been traumatised, can struggle, can withdraw. I mean, in extreme cases, they may be dissociating into some place in themselves that they learned to go into, say, in childhood, in order to cope. A place where they simply had to reinforce the view that they were a bad or difficult person. Now this gets triggered and this in turn sets off a set of behaviours that reinforce that belief, which could include non-compliance with those who are trying to help them. I'm afraid I've heard the phrase, "mad, bad, or sad" too often. People need time to trust and time to feel heard and understood. They need time for the uniqueness of their experience – yes, of course it might take the same form as other's – but it is their experience, and they have their felt meanings associated with it.' Carla sighed and shook her head. 'I guess I have strong views, but they aren't just ideas I have in isolation, I have worked with people who have mental health diagnoses, and I know what I have heard them say about their treatment. Why do people go into psychotic states? How many "voices" are simply "dissociative states" emerging, or even "configuration within the self" that have particularly strong identities finding a way of being heard?'

Configurations within self (Mearns and Thorne, 2000) are discrete sets of thoughts, feelings and behaviours that develop through the experience of life. They emerge in response to a range of experiences including the process of introjection and the symbolisation of experiences, as well as in response to dissonant self-experience within the person's structure of self. They can also exist in what Mearns terms as 'growthful' and 'not for growth' configurations, the former seemingly providing a focus for the actualising tendency, the latter those that seek to block change because of its potential for disrupting the current order within the structure of self (Mearns and Thorne, 2000). The self, then, is seen as a constellation of configurations, with the individual moving between them and living through them in response to experience.

Mearns suggests that these 'parts' or 'configurations' interrelate 'like a family, with an individual variety of dynamics'. As within any 'system', change in one area will impact on the functioning of the system. He therefore comments that 'when the interrelationship of configurations changes, it is not that we are left with something entirely new: we have the same "parts" as before, but some which may have been subservient before are stronger, others which were judged adversely are accepted, some which were in self-negating conflict have come to respect each other, and overall the parts have achieved constructive integration with the energy release which arises from such fusion'. (Mearns, 1999, pp. 147–8)

Warner (2002) writes that 'dissociated experiences ... are a great deal more personified than ordinary mood states or even "configurations" ' and that 'dissociated process seems to arise almost exclusively as a response to early childhood trauma'. She goes on to say that these dissociated parts 'seem to emerge when trauma memories are pressing to the surface'. (Warner, pp. 158–63)

'That's an interesting point. As you say, certain psychotic experiences are perhaps the effect of psychological processes that may be rooted in unrecognised trauma, or in particularly well-defined configurational states that have developed as part of the normal psychological process. It seems to require, though, that whether we are talking about a "configurational part" or a "dissociative part", in order for its presence to manifest through what gets labelled as a psychotic episode, it had to be very well defined as a discrete entity, with a strong identity within the structure of self.'

'I really think that the person-centred approach has a lot to offer in understanding these kinds of experience. I really do. And yes, as I say, of course there are people for whom there is a need for chemical treatment – long term or short term – to address a chemical imbalance, a genuine medical condition. But I wonder just how many are being treated long term through chemical intervention for states of mind that are experientially induced and need an experiential process to resolve them? I come back to my albeit simplistic belief that people damaged by unhealthy and abusive relational experiences stand the best chance of resolving them through experiencing healthy relational experiences. And I think Rogers, when he emphasised his six necessary and sufficient conditions for constructive personality change (Rogers, 1957), is saying something that should underpin all treatment. I really do.'

'That there is a fundamental quality of relationship that is necessary, but clearly not always sufficient given that there could be chemical imbalance that has an organic basis.' William was careful with his wording, aware that there was and had seemed always to have been this discussion since Rogers formulated this idea as to whether the conditions were both necessary and sufficient.

'I agree. But it is a difficult area, and, yes, the approach can and does help people with mental health problems. And yes, medication helps and is necessary in

some cases, but the need for a quality and healthy relationship with people, with those who are offering treatment, has to be important. I can't see how it cannot be. Any healthcare professional, it seems to me, needs to apply Rogers' principles – I think of them as "principles of effective human relationship" – accurate empathy, congruence, warm acceptance of the client, and all communicated to and received accurately by the client because there is an established psychological contact – however minimal that might be, at least to start with.'
'And the factor of it being minimal can be particularly relevant here.'
Carla nodded. 'Yes, think of the pre-therapy work that is being done. This is an important development and application of the person-centred approach. I am thinking not only of the factor of psychological contact, but also that of the different aspects of empathy that the pre-therapy system defines.'

In the pre-therapy model, a distinction is drawn between 'empathy' as described earlier, and 'empathic contact'. In a situation in which 'the therapist does not know the client's inner frame of reference', then 'the empathy is for the client's effort at developing coherent experience and expression, perhaps a form of consolidating the self-formative tendency during these primitive phases of therapy'. Prouty goes on to suggest a second level of empathy which he defines as being for 'the concrete particularity of behavioural expression', in other words, 'not focused on the generalized "essence" of meaning, but on the literal expressive behaviour'. The third level of empathy which he then suggests concerns 'the increase in psychotic expression as a function of pre-therapy'. It is worth quoting verbatim what he has to say regarding this as it is clearly a view that many mental health professionals would find challenging: 'The client needs to get worse before she can get better. The therapist needs to be empathic to an increase in delusional and hallucinatory expression, as well as to an increase in bizarre communication (strange body language, postures, language disturbance, etc.). This means being empathic to the lived experience of the psychosis itself. This is, of course, the opposite of behavioural and chemical management.' (Prouty, 2002, p. 63)

William agreed. 'OK, so I know I started this discussion, and I think it is valuable and important to make these connections in our understanding of the application of our theoretical framework. I am also becoming increasingly mindful as I sit here of Fareeda, where she is in all of this, and whether you need time to process your responses to her during our time now.' He had noted a sense of Fareeda becoming less present. It wasn't that he was not attending to Carla, or believing that the focus of their exploration was important, it was, but he felt that the client was being left out of the loop, as it were, and felt a need to invite her presence back into the exploration that was taking place between Carla and himself.

'I'm feeling more and more for Fareeda. Since our last supervision session I think I have felt generally more sensitive and open to her. The issues we discussed last time I feel I have been able to put to one side, and I feel I am much more in touch with her, particularly after she shared some Islamic prayers and sayings with me. Ali's poem also touched me deeply, he has felt more present too. It was a poem about hopelessness, really, very powerful. And in a way this brought me more into the sessions. I think it is something about being a mother myself, perhaps we became two mothers rather than counsellor–client, to some degree. Whether that's OK or not, I'm not sure, but perhaps as I think about it now that is the nature of what occurred. This has enabled me to empathise I think more fully, not just with Fareeda, but with the situation that she finds herself in.'

William nodded and wanted to explore this further. 'So, the sense of your being a mother, how specifically does that help you? How might that affect you as compared to a counsellor who, say, isn't a mother, or a parent even, for instance? She might have been seen by a male counsellor.'

Carla thought. 'Interesting question, that. What do I bring as a mother? Maybe there is something that makes my . . .', Carla paused, 'I'm not sure how best to describe this . . .'

'Well, maybe just think out loud and see what emerges.'

Carla nodded as she sought to clarify for herself what she felt in response to William's question. It was a good one, and she was aware of how it was really focusing herself on exactly what she was offering, and how, in a sense, that was linked to her own identity.

'I think that it has something to do with how I can be, how I may respond. I think I can come from a place of knowing from my own experience of what being a mother can be like, and yet, as we know, all experiences are unique, with each person taking their own meaning. So it isn't like I'm an expert on Fareeda's experience because of my own. It's not that at all. But it's like, well, maybe it affects something of the tone of what I say, maybe the part of me that if you like is associated with my mothering experience somehow reaches out to the client who has their own similar, yet unique, identity as a mother.' Carla paused to reflect on what she had said. Did that sound right? Was it what she wanted to say?

Wiliam reflected her words. He didn't add his view or opinion, simply allowed Carla to hear what she had said. 'So, the part of you that is associated with being a mother somehow reaches out to the part of the client that is their identity as a mother? That what you mean?'

The words weren't exactly her own but, yes, it was something like that. 'Yes, and I'm back thinking of configurations here. If we think of person-centred theory then yes, why shouldn't there be some kind of relationship created between parts of me and parts of my client? If we take the idea that the structure of self is made up of parts, some more discrete identities than others, then why shouldn't the fact that within me is present a "mother part" have significance in some way for clients who either have their own version of the same part . . .' Carla paused as another idea struck her. 'But it's more than that, isn't it? Because if I work with a client who, as a son or daughter, has their sense of self shaped by their experience of being mothered, they will perhaps be responding to the part of me that is the mother. Oh, this is complex, isn't it?'

William nodded. 'Yes, it is, and yet there is also a fundamental simplicity, and it all comes back to our congruence. Can I as a person in the counselling role be fully aware of myself to the point that I can recognise all the different parts of me and understand my own process in response to what the client is presenting to me?'

Carla took a deep breath. 'For me that emphasises even more the challenge of working to a theory in which we use ourselves, where the therapeutic process is very much centred on the relationship, on how the counsellor and client relate to one another.'

'Mhmm, so the mother part in you will have its own associated thoughts, feelings, behaviours, yes? The mother part in you, the fact that it is present and the form it takes, will convey something to the client.'

'And it may be quite subtle, mightn't it? I mean, it might simply affect the way that I speak. I may not need to disclose whether or not I am a mother, but simply my presence as a mother, how I am because of my experience, may convey something to the client who will then take from that, well, whatever they take from it. I can't define what that will be.'

'So, yes, something is conveyed . . .' William empathised with Carla and left his response in the air, being aware that whilst they had acknowledged something was conveyed exactly what hadn't been identified.

Carla was still trying to identify the illusive 'something'. What did she bring into her relationship with Fareeda because she was a mother? What did the mothering part of her contain? 'I don't think I've voiced this to Fareeda, I'm not sure, but I don't think so. But it seems to me that what she pulls from me, and maybe this is from the mothering part of me, is a real sense of her devotion – no, hearing myself say that I know I haven't used that word. But it is a sense that I have, and I can relate to that, of her dedication, yes, that's an important word, her dedication to her son. I think that links with my experience as well. As a mother I know I will put my child first, I know that. It's what I do.'

'So devotion, dedication, both resonate with the mother in you?'

'Very much so. I have reflected on how I would be in her situation. Not in the session, but wondered how would I be? Would I be any different if my son had similar problems? Would I see them as a problem, first of all? And I'm sure I would. I'd want to help, be there for him, help him to get the help he needs. And even if I don't say this I am sure that the mother part of me brings a certain, I don't know, I nearly said authenticity, but I don't mean that. You don't have to have been a mother to be authentic. But it brings a certain – I'm almost tempted to say solidarity, but perhaps I mean something more in the way of commonality.'

'A commonality . . . , of experience, you mean?'

'Something like that, a kind of commonality of . . .' Carla paused. A commonality of what? 'It's something about recognising that a part of me has developed out of an experience or experiences that have some link to that which has been experienced, or is being experienced, by the client.'

That sounded clear to William. 'So, and these are my words and meaning, the commonality of an experience enables you to access that part of your own experience that has similarities, and I am also aware of thinking that there is something about context here as well. That your own experience puts you in touch with the context of mothering, in the sense that whilst you have your version of this, and so does the client, the generalism of mothering is a commonality even though it will probably take different forms.'

Carla was nodding. 'Yes, yes, that helps me. And this brings me to realise that it has enabled me to move beyond the differences – the ethnic context – which was present early in our relationship.'

William smiled. 'The question remains, however, was that dealt with, or was it put aside by the emergence of the mothering commonality providing the primary point of contact between parts of yourselves?'

Time was running out in the supervision session and Carla immediately recognised that what had now emerged was important and something she needed to think about. It wasn't a perspective that she had considered before. Yes, I have an identity as a mother, as a woman, and those can become the focus for my connecting with Fareeda, but where does her experience as a Muslim come in, because I don't have a sense of self that has developed within that experience?

Carla and William felt they had a great deal to reflect on after the session had ended. The idea that the structure of self was made up of parts had enormous implications for person-centred theory and the more they thought about it, the more significant those implications were. It left Carla more aware of her own complexity and the sense that she needed, somehow, to be aware within counselling sessions of how the many parts of her were reacting or responding to her clients. She had the image of all these non-verbal dialogues taking place, some of which became actual verbal dialogues. It left her feeling quite quiet and humbled as she pondered on the vastness of the process, the complexity and yet, as well, the fact that it was, in essence, a matter of communication and relationship. The trick, if there was one, was to be aware of the communications that were taking place (or not taking place) and shaping the quality of the therapeutic relationship.

Counselling session 5: Wednesday 15th April – the discharge meeting and Fareeda's hopes for Ali's treatment

Fareeda had found the discharge meeting quite daunting. It had taken place in a small room and there seemed to be a number of people involved.

'There was the psychiatrist, another doctor I think, and a nurse from the ward, there was Desmond who is a nurse from the drug team, myself and, of course, Ali. Oh, and someone taking notes. I took along a statement and made sure copies were given out.'

Carla nodded, wondering whether Fareeda would want to describe how she felt or how it was received, or both, or something else. She maintained her person-centred focus and allowed her space to continue as she wanted to.

'They had already decided that basically the problems Ali had were a reaction to the cannabis, and so the idea was for Desmond to see Ali.' She shook her head. 'I know it's not just the cannabis, but they weren't accepting that. Yes, what just happened was probably connected to it, but not the past. I tried to tell them, and Ali tried to tell them as well, but they seemed – at least the consultant seemed – so sure and, well, everyone seemed to just agree with him. I really didn't feel heard although I did read out my statement.'

Carla noted the worn expression on Fareeda's face. 'Must have got to you. You look pretty worn down by it all.'

'Yes, but I spoke to Desmond afterwards and, well, he seemed more open. Said he didn't like those meetings, and that he appreciated what I was saying. It seems that although he works for the adult drug service, he has a lot of experience of working with younger people. He's not a therapist though, and I made the point that I felt that therapy was what Ali needed. I wanted him to be able to make sense of his experience, of being able to work in a therapeutic way.'

'Mhmm, that's the bit that I know you feel passionate about.'

'Yes, I do, but, well, it seems like that's not available. At least, it is but there will be a wait. They don't employ therapists in the drug team at the moment but they do have voluntary placements for experienced therapists who want to develop their practice of working with clients using substances. They also have voluntary counsellors who are in training, but Desmond felt that given what Ali had experienced, he could probably be seen by one of the more experienced counsellors. But he would assess him first and, if Ali agreed, then he could set up the counselling once a slot was available.'

'Structured counselling' should be available to all who require this as part of their package of treatment for drug and alcohol problems. It may not always be available within a particular drug team, however. Often different treatment responses are located within statutory and non-statutory services. The 'Models of care' system for drug service provision attempts to ensure that clients with substance misuse problems can access a range of services within their area (National Treatment Agency, 2002; Bryant-Jefferies, 2004). An issue for the counselling profession, however, is to what degree their profession is recognised as part of the core services for working with clients for whom substance misuse behaviour requires therapeutic work. Coupled to this is a secondary issue, that of competency for working in this area. The act of substance misuse is complex in itself, and when you add to this the factor of potential mental health problems and traumatic experiences associated with and/or as causative factors in the choice to use substances, the counsellor will need to have an appropriate level of competence. Also, there must be in place the quality of therapeutic supervision that will be required as part of the process of ensuring safe practice.

'So, some form of therapeutic counselling will be available, but there will be a wait?'
'Yes, and Desmond will be what I think he said was a "keyworker". He'd see Ali as well to see how he was progressing and liaise with the counsellor. Ali may also see someone else who would be responsible for overseeing what he was being offered and his progress. He wasn't sure who that would be. Some other person – a "care co-ordinator" I think, though this hasn't been definitely agreed upon. Seems a lot of people involved.'
Carla was aware that it could seem like that. She just hoped Ali would relate well to the people involved. In her experience, the more people on a case, the greater the risk that the client could get confused, or get caught up in an endless cycle of appointments. She hoped the counsellor would be allowed to get on with the therapeutic work and the other contacts would be minimal, but that probably reflected her own prejudices.

Under the 'Models of care' system for drug treatment, clients may have a keyworker within a treatment service as well as a care co-ordinator outside of the service; the latter co-ordinating treatment and care in line with care planning and, where necessary, involving more than one service in providing treatment, or co-ordinating the movement of the client through services. This might seem excessive, but the idea is to ensure clear lines of liaison and integrated pathways of care with treatment response being more client-centred, rather than a 'one size fits all' approach. This system is likely to be reviewed, however, as there is confusion over the role of the care co-ordinator. Not everyone needs a care co-ordinator, only those with complex needs and difficulties.

'Mhmm, feels like too many people?'
'Well, I don't know enough to know if that's the case, but it does seem like a lot, although in another way I'm just glad that Ali is going to get attention, and hopefully it will work out.' She took a deep breath. 'I couldn't face going through all of this again.'
'No, you want it to work out and for Ali to be helped.'
Fareeda nodded. 'So I guess things have worked out OK. At the moment Ali is seeing Desmond quite a lot, seems to be in touch every day. It's helping to get Ali out. He's not getting the strange ideas in his head, and he tells me he's not smoking the cannabis. He's not in his room as much; that's a good sign, I think.'

'So, you are feeling a little more positive?'

'I think so, but I suppose I'm still aware that Ali's mood has been erratic in the past and, well, just wonder how he will react if that happens again.'

'Yes, knowing what that can be like . . .'

'It's just that, well, I know things can change. Guess I'm a worrier.'

Carla smiled. 'You're his mother, of course you will be concerned. But hopefully his stability will be good for you as well.'

'Yes, and I suppose that will happen. But at the moment I'm still anxious about how he is, how he will be when I come home, you know?'

Carla nodded. 'That anxiety is something that has been with you for a while, it won't pass overnight.'

'I guess it will take time, but at least I feel Ali is getting help. He seems to get on well with Desmond. I ask Ali what they talk about and he just says "stuff". He hasn't said much more about what they talk about precisely, but maybe he will in the future. I gather, though, that he may be offered a place at a group run by another service. He did mention that to me. We do seem to be talking more. It's early days, isn't it? I keep saying my prayers. Maybe they are being answered.' Fareeda looked into Carla's eyes, it seemed like she was seeking some kind of acknowledgement from Carla that she felt that her prayers were being answered.

'Maybe. As you say, he is getting help, it sounds like he is getting on well with Desmond. Let's hope it is a time of change – for everyone.' Carla knew she hadn't really empathised, and she knew her 'for everyone' was pointed not only at Fareeda but also at her husband, Chris.

'I hope so, Carla, I really do. I don't know how much more I could have taken before it all blew up. Ali was so weird and the thought that he might end up like that again . . .' Fareeda paused, the images of how it had been were very clear, as were the feelings that they aroused within her. 'I don't think he really appreciates how ill he was. I have told him and I know they did on the ward once he was more stable. He said that it wasn't so much weird to him, at the time it made sense, but it was scary in the sense that he knew he believed, totally, what he was thinking about people spying on him. He knows he has to keep off the cannabis. Everyone at the discharge meeting was very clear on that. The psychiatrist explained how some people were more susceptible than others and that Ali was one of those people for whom cannabis was bad news. They didn't say anything about the different types, I guess they didn't want to encourage him to try the weaker stuff. They were clear in saying it needed to be avoided because he clearly reacted badly to it. I don't think that message is broadcast enough. It's all too much of a laugh for young people, a buzz, but they shouldn't need to have to have a chemical to feel good. I know that, well, Ali has had his mood swings and maybe that makes it different and more difficult, I'm sure it does. But so many people use drugs these days – and alcohol – I don't go into town any more in the evenings on some nights, it's just not safe. And yet it just becomes more and more available. We were brought up to avoid drinking alcohol. Whether that's the answer, I'm not sure.'

'That was because of your parents' religious beliefs?'

'Yes, and I think it left me with a sense that alcohol's not really important. Yes, I drink occasionally. My parents still don't and I guess never will. And that's fine, it's how they choose to be. But I feel like there is something in me, something in-built, that just isn't attracted to the idea of drinking heavily. There's no attraction for me. I'd rather do other things.'

'Mhmm, other things that give you, what, good feelings?'

Fareeda nodded. 'And I realise I need more of that. I can see how I've been so caught up with Ali that I haven't maybe given myself time for things for me.'

Carla smiled. Yes, she thought to herself, it felt good to hear that. 'More time for things for you. That feels good.' She kept her empathic response short and to the point.

'I think it'll take time, but I do need to do other things. I'm still not clear where my marriage is going. Some of the things that have happened as a result of how Ali is, well, I don't know whether it will last, and whether I really want it to last. But I have to think of Adam as well, and what will be best for him. He gets on well with his dad and maybe I need to accept things for a little longer and, well, maybe things will improve.' As she spoke Fareeda knew that whilst she did want what was best for her sons, she also knew that she wasn't happy in the marriage. What did Allah want her to do? The question remained, unanswered. She would do her best, do her duty. 'I want to be there for my sons. That's important to me. At some point I want to try and encourage Chris to come to couples counselling.' She shook her head, feeling it was hard to imagine how this might occur. 'We need help to talk, I think.'

'So, time for you, but also time to be there for your sons, and a sense of needing to find ways to help you and Chris talk.'

Fareeda nodded. That summed it all up pretty clearly. She took a deep breath. 'It feels uncertain at the moment, but I need to be optimistic, somehow.'

Carla nodded. Her thoughts momentarily went back to the supervision session. It struck her how Fareeda the wife was another part of herself that would impact on Carla the wife as well. She smiled to herself as she thought of the complexity of the two of them sitting in the counselling room, and yet the simplicity as well. What a paradox, she thought to herself. The simplicity of two people sitting together and communicating, and yet the complexity of what contributes to that process. Uncertainty and optimism, yes, that summed up life. We never knew what was coming next but somehow we had to keep hope alive.

'Yes, that sounds really important.' Carla smiled as she spoke. 'And I'm struck by the simplicity of us sitting here, two women, and yet the complexity with all the issues that are present, and the differences between us, and the similarities as well.'

Fareeda smiled back. It did feel like a weight had been lifted, at least a little bit. It was complex and yet the simplicity of having someone to talk to, someone who really listened, just seemed so valuable. So much had happened since she had begun seeing Carla. It hadn't been easy at the start and then things had got worse with Ali, but now, well, now things seemed to be changing for the better. The thought of Ali getting worse again wasn't something she wanted to contemplate, although she knew that within her the fear of that happening was present. But she would try and push it aside and get on with her life. Her family was important to her – in truth the most important part of her life. She was on God's earth to be a mother, that was how she felt, and she wanted to be a good one. She felt tears in her eyes as she had these thoughts.

The session continued with Fareeda talking about the importance to her of being a good mother. She spoke a little more about her own background, her own childhood, her parents. It somehow felt to Carla as though Fareeda was becoming even more present to her, and she appreciated this and told her that this was what she was experiencing. It was genuine and Fareeda experienced that genuineness. It felt good. It encouraged her to share more. It was a definite moving on in their relationship.

Towards the end of the session Fareeda asked how many more sessions she needed. Carla indicated that really it was up to her and asked why she had asked the question at this time?

'I don't want to stop, I'm finding it really helpful. I look forward to coming. It frees me up, somehow, and helps me unload. And it helps me think about things. Talking about my background, my family, feeling you listening, it felt good, and it makes me realise how much I want that feeling, and somehow I have lost something of that.'

'I'm aware of how important family is to you, Fareeda, and yes, the feeling you get from talking the way you have, and from being listened to, it's a good feeling.'

'But I have lost it, though maybe I can find it again.' Fareeda needed to mention the losing it again, felt that she needed Carla to hear that.

'Mhmm, lost but maybe it is there to be found again.'

'So, how many sessions so far, five, isn't it?'

Carla nodded, hoping that Fareeda wouldn't want to stop – she enjoyed the sessions, and yet she knew that she must let Fareeda make her own choices. There were always reasons to hang on to clients, the counsellor could always identify work to be done, but it was up to the client in her view to judge what she wanted to work on, and when. Some people wanted long-term therapy, others to dip in and out as problems or issues arose.

'Well, it feels good for me, and that's what I need at the moment.'

'I'm really pleased. I feel good working with you, and I want to offer whatever I can as you move along this part of life's journey.' Ouch, Carla thought, that felt a little bit like sickly 'counsellor-speak'.

The session drew to a close. The relationship would be ongoing. Exactly how long for, only time would tell. Carla watched Fareeda head out of the door and closed it behind her. She wanted to be optimistic, like Fareeda, and she knew that realistically things may not be as smooth as she would hope. But perhaps it would all work out. She sat down and reflected on the counselling process so far. Five sessions and yet so much had happened for Fareeda. And the counselling relationship had moved on as well. It felt as though the relationship was developing, as though more aspects of Fareeda were becoming present which, in turn, drew more of Carla into the relationship as well. That felt satisfying as well as important.

She had learned a lot about herself these past few weeks, but she was still aware of that comment in her last supervision session. Yes, maybe she had connected with Fareeda as a mother, and as a woman, perhaps, but maybe there were other areas that did need further work. Perhaps the mother connection was giving her a false sense of the completeness of their counselling relationship. No, completeness seemed too big a word for it. They had found an area of connection but there were other areas to be explored as well, if that was what Fareeda wanted – or perhaps what her actualising tendency wanted to emphasise. Carla shook her head as she contemplated this. She loved the idea of an actualising tendency within everyone, a kind of living process – or was it a process of living – that urged the person towards a fuller and more satisfying experience of life. She smiled as she thought about how she, and everyone, goes about their life, doing what they do, making the choices that they make, quite unaware of this internal process. Funny old thing, life, she thought to herself. We think we know so much and yet we seem to understand so little. She began to write her notes for the session.

As she left, Fareeda stood for a moment in the driveway and took a deep breath. She had heard the door close behind her. Somehow that seemed to be symbolic of something. Such a little everyday thing, and yet . . . It wasn't that the door to her counselling had closed, but it was like something inside her perhaps was closing, maybe some part of her life. She hoped so. She thought of Ali. He was different now and she saw glimpses of the son she knew, the son that she knew he could be, and she just prayed it would last. She said a short prayer under her breath. The sun was shining. Life still had its difficulties and, yes, uncertainties, she knew that, but somehow she felt stronger, more able to cope. Something about coming and talking, and being listened to, being heard. In a way it was a strange experience and yet somehow not so strange. It felt natural. She walked slowly to her car, still deep in thought. She hoped Ali was going to be OK, and she hoped that she and Chris would resolve the difficulties that had arisen between them. She unlocked the door and put her bag on the passenger seat. She paused to switch on her mobile phone. There was a voice message. It was Adam, sounding very anxious – he wasn't at school that day. 'Mum, can you come home as soon as possible. Ali's acting weird again.'

Summary

Fareeda describes the discharge meeting for Ali and what is being set up. Also her hope that he will now get the help that he needs. She also talks about her own past and her parents, and it feels to Carla as though Fareeda becomes a little more present to her. Fareeda communicates how helpful the sessions are and of her intention to continue with them. Carla reflects on the session in the light of her experience in supervision of exploring the idea that people relate to each other through parts of themselves that have some kind of resonance with each other.

Points for discussion

- How are you feeling at the end of counselling session 5? What reactions are present within you?
- The notion of parts communicating with each other – reflect on this from your own experience. What are your conclusions as to the correctness of this idea?
- How do you respond to the issues raised in supervision session 2? What implications do they have for your own practice?
- What other factors might you have wanted to have brought to supervision had you been Carla?
- Is William an effective supervisor based on what you have read? Why do you reach your conclusion?
- What issues would you expect Fareeda will need to deal with in the coming sessions over and above those related directly to Ali?
- Critically analyse Carla's application of person-centred theory to her counselling work with Fareeda across the five sessions.
- Write your own notes for counselling session 5.

PART 2

Her son begins his own counselling process

CHAPTER 6

Desmond had told Ali that the counselling could start the following week. Ali was in two minds. Since coming out of the hospital things had not been easy and three weeks had passed. To start with, all had been fine, but some of the old feelings and thoughts had returned – feelings of suspicion and the sense that people were looking at him and knew all about him – and he'd smoked some cannabis. It had made him feel better. But it had changed his behaviour and it was this that had alerted his brother. Too bright that kid, was what Ali thought. But anyway, he'd been seen by the mental health team for a follow-up not long after they had discharged him from the hospital and they had told him to stop using cannabis, that it was causing him problems. Ali knew that he smoked to try and stop his thoughts, to quell the discomfort and unease inside himself, but they weren't prepared to accept that. They just kept telling him to stop the cannabis and to take his medication. Well, he was trying but he missed the feelings he got from using the cannabis.

Ali had previously been assessed by the drug team. They were also encouraging him to take his medication, but they seemed to go about it in a different way. They seemed to accept that he was using to make himself feel easier, but also told him that sometimes whilst it could help to begin with, after time it could make things worse. They also talked more about the different kinds of cannabis and just how much stronger the 'skunk' cannabis was compared to the pot he'd been smoking in the past. He had to agree that what he'd smoked more recently had been the stronger, 'skunk' cannabis. The trouble was, as he told them, you weren't really sure what you were getting when you bought it, and you didn't want to waste it.

The upshot of it all was that he was now being seen regularly by Desmond. He had also been seen by the doctor at the drug service and they had agreed to arrange for him to have counselling. They had long recognised that as a service they needed to broaden their work, and as a result had developed an on-site counselling service. Whilst Ali would have a keyworker within the service – Desmond was a community psychiatric nurse and so could work with and monitor Ali's mental health and his drug use, using cognitive-behavioural therapy and motivational interviewing techniques – he would also be offered person-centred therapeutic counselling on a regular basis.

It seems to be a reasonable package of treatment, offering the client keyworking to monitor his mental health and to provide some cognitive-behavioural input to help him manage his difficulties, and at the same time to offer a therapeutic counselling approach to give the client a different experience and an opportunity to explore, at greater depth perhaps, the underlying issues and experiences that might be fuelling his psychotic episodes.

So, Ali was standing outside the building where the drug service was located. It was a modern-looking building, and didn't look like it had been used for more than a couple of years or so. He thought about what he was doing. The thought of yet another person to talk to. Desmond had been quite encouraging about the counselling, and said that the counsellor could help him to understand himself more and maybe talk about things that perhaps he had wanted to talk about but had never been quite able to. Desmond had a sense that there was more to Ali's problem than simply drug use, and whilst he recognised that his mental state could be diagnosed as psychotic, the culture of the unit was not to rush into medicalising his problem too quickly, and rather to take a more psychological view. So when someone was referred with psychotic symptoms they would begin from the premise that the client was creating what, from the outside, might seem like a delusional world, but for the client was perhaps reasonable and somehow in keeping with something within their structure of self. It was an innovative approach in many ways, trying not to rush into pathological viewpoints.

So the decision for Ali to receive counselling was in order for him to explore himself and perhaps feel able, in time, to open up whatever was present within him that caused the delusional states to take the form that they did. Their belief was that by so doing, there was a likelihood that the client could reprocess what they were experiencing and perhaps put aside the need for the delusional experiences, or if not, accept them and relate to them in a way that they became less disruptive to the individual's life and those around them. If this proved ineffective, if the delusional states were out of control and/or there was clear risk to the client or others, then they would use medication.

Counselling session 1: Tuesday 5th May – counselling begins, the client is restless, ends with a relaxation visualisation

Ali was sitting in the counselling room with Charlotte, his counsellor. She had explained to him the nature and purpose of counselling and he had sat quietly listening to her. At least, he didn't say much but he found it hard to stay settled.

He tended to move around a lot in the chair anyway; he hadn't really felt able to be still for a long while. In fact, he was now quite oblivious to his restlesness when he wasn't smoking the dope. He wasn't sure that he trusted Charlotte. She wasn't like Desmond. Yeah, OK, she seemed to know her stuff, seemed friendly, but, well, Desmond he sort of respected. Not that he told Desmond much about himself, not about his past anyway. Well, that didn't feel comfortable. That was the past, anyway, his problems were now. At least, everyone said his problems were now.

At some level Ali knew they were right, but there were times as well when he knew he was OK, that he could handle things, that the dope wasn't a problem. He thought of Desmond again, his face with that big grin. Yeah, he felt good with him. Was it his colour? He didn't know. He tended to feel a bit more guarded with white folk. Charlotte was white. He just accepted that was how he was, coming from a mixed-race background. He reckoned that was the way anyone was who was of mixed-race or black. He'd learned as a child not to trust white kids. They'd bullied him, picked on him, taunted him about his colour. He learned later that that wasn't always the case, and although he didn't have strong views now, he knew that he had a sense of an allegiance to people of colour. And deep down, he wasn't really sure how much he could trust white people.

In making these comments there is no intention to stereotype. This is simply the character of one person which has developed out of his own set of difficult and damaging experiences in life, a character that will also have been shaped by cultural influences and expectations.

So, he sat, withdrawing from Charlotte. It wasn't exactly a conscious process, it was one of the ways he had learned to cope with situations – and new people – that he felt unsure about. Charlotte was talking about confidentiality. 'What you say is confidential but there is a limit to that, and I want to be clear with you about this.'

Ali nodded, 'Yeah, OK.' Desmond had talked to him about confidentiality as well. He didn't say anything to Charlotte, let her keep talking. She was telling him when she would have to break confidentiality. He was getting bored. 'Yeah, Desmond told me about that.'

'OK, and was what he said similar to what I'm saying?'

Ali nodded. It all sounded the same to him.

'And with the limits to confidentiality?'

'If I threaten to harm myself, or someone else, that kind of stuff.'

'Including planned threats, or, as I say to everyone, people planning acts of terrorism.'

Ali felt himself react. Desmond hadn't said that, just said about threats to harm others. Why was she saying this to him? He wasn't devout at all, but he did have a real sense of his Muslim 'brothers' who were out there in the world being treated badly. He felt for them. Yeah, he was no bomber, but hell, people got a right to fight for their freedom. It irritated him hearing her talk like that. What did she know? What did she know about the shit lives his 'brothers' had to put up with around the world? He felt himself feeling even less like talking to her.

Comments made can so easily create barriers if they haven't been thought through. Charlotte's comment regarding terrorism needs to be set in the current context. It is a confidentiality issue and it does need to be mentioned. However, it is a topic that could be misunderstood by clients, or provoke a reaction that might become a barrier to the formation of a therapeutic relationship. Yet it is important to stress how it is something that is explained to everyone, though better still if the nature and limits of confidentiality are available in a leaflet to be given to every client, which can minimise the risk of a client thinking they are, for whatever reason, being singled out. This is even more important when a client has evidenced paranoid tendencies. Everyone should be treated equally. Counsellors do not sit down with a new client and immediately begin anticipating that the client has an intent to do serious harm to others. But the reality is that there are limits to confidentiality that the client needs to understand, and this is one of them. It forms part of the counselling contract. Of course, the counsellor has no control over a client's reaction. There will always be clients who, for all kinds of reasons, choose not to continue with counselling because of a concern – maybe not expressed – about the limits of confidentiality. Child protection issues can be another such area.

'The bottom line for me is about helping you to keep yourself well and safe.' Charlotte was aware she was talking too much. She was anxious. She had worked with some younger people, but she wasn't really at ease. She knew she was talking from her nerves and she needed to slow down and give Ali some space.

Ali looked at the ground. Fancy words, he thought, just fancy words. 'Yeah, well, I don't want medication. Fed up with taking the pills, you know? Not interested in pills. I like to smoke, that's what makes me feel cool, yeah? I just want to feel normal, you know?'

'Normal?' Charlotte responded in such a way so as to empathise that she heard Ali, and also invite clarification.

'Yeah, normal, you know, smoke a little dope, have friends, listen to music and, yeah, spend a bit of money, have a good time. I just want to take it easy.'

'Mhmm.' Charlotte nodded. She accepted Ali's priorities for a normal life, noting that the dope had been the first item on his list of components for a normal life. And whilst his keyworker may have picked up on that and focused on it, to help Ali explore what his dope use meant to him, and maybe look for opportunities to motivate him to change, using motivational interviewing techniques (Miller and Rollnick, 1991), her role as a person-centred therapeutic counsellor was to accept how Ali needed to be and help him explore whatever was most important to him.

'Mhmm, that sounds pretty clear to me, Ali, smoke a bit of dope, friends, music, spend a bit of money, take it easy. Sounds good to you, huh.' She added the sounds good, sensing that this was how it felt for Ali and wanting to empathise with her sensed perception of how he viewed this ideal 'normal'.

'Yeah. So, what do we talk about?'

'What's on your mind?' Charlotte realised that her open response had probably directed Ali more towards a focus on his thinking than his feelings. She acknowledged to herself that maybe that wasn't appropriate, although she also knew that what she had said was kind of a colloquial response and so may not be taken that way by Ali.

'Don't know, really, feel like I want to feel a bit more settled, you know?' He was still moving around in the chair, unable to be still, not that he was trying to be.

'In yourself, do you mean, or in parts of your life?'

'Yeah, everywhere. I don't know, I feel on edge, you know,' he tightened his lips and clenched his teeth behind them. 'Just feel kind of, you know, can't sort of settle. Keep feeling jumpy, can't settle. Desmond says that's the effect of not smoking the skunk, you know? Maybe he's right. The medication doesn't help that. Still feel uptight.' He moved around in his seat again.

Charlotte raised her hands a little in front of her as she spoke. 'Like, yeah, have to keep moving.' She moved her hands as she spoke and moved herself in her chair.

'Yeah, that's right. And I can't sleep. Shit, I lay there for hours at night. Listen to music, end up falling asleep but it's usually nearly morning.'

'So, you spend the nights listening to music?'

'And thinking. Does my head in, thoughts going round and round. Dope stops it. The medication sort of does a bit, but not the same.'

Charlotte was aware of Ali's background and what had brought him into the drug team for help. So her immediate wonder was what thoughts were going round in his head, and were they the thoughts that spun out of control. But at the same time she didn't want to be directive, she accepted wholeheartedly the non-directive nature of the person-centred approach. She saw herself as being there to facilitate Ali in resolving conflicts and incongruencies within himself, but for this to occur she knew she needed not only to be able to communicate empathy and unconditional positive regard, but also her own authenticity. She worked at the unit because she valued their philosophy. She wanted to understand Ali, help him make sense of himself if that was what he wanted to do. Help him resolve the difficulties that beset him if that was what he wanted to address.

'So, yeah, thoughts going round and round in your head.' She emphasised it by speaking slowly.

'Yeah. Gets to me. Really does my head in.'

'Yeah, and I'm not going to say that I can imagine how it must be because I don't know what it must be like. But I'd like to help you make sense of it.' Charlotte was totally genuine in what she said.

She knew only too well that it was pointless to simply try and say to someone that you understood. What did that convey? Chances are the client would simply feel fobbed off. Better to be open and honest. Yes, she could appreciate that it must be a problem for Ali but she had no idea what it was like to experience his thoughts in his head, going round and round, night after night.

'Mhmm.' Ali stayed silent. He didn't want to talk about the stuff at night. Some of it was stupid, he knew that, but sometimes it also seemed real as well, and that was scary. He'd lie there listening for sounds, and he'd hear them, and convince himself it was somebody out there trying to spy on him. He knew it was stupid, at least he knew it now. Sometimes he didn't. Sometimes it was for real. He was sure of it. But then he'd tell himself not to be stupid, remind himself what they'd said in the hospital about his thoughts, his paranoia. Having a word for it didn't help him much.

Charlotte sat feeling suddenly cut off from Ali, as if he had stepped away from her psychologically.

'I don't want to go back in hospital again.' He spoke quite quietly. He was shaking his head and pulling a face.

'Don't want to go back in hospital?' Again, she added a hint of questioning to her empathic response.

Ali continued to shake his head. 'Crazy people in there, shouting, screaming, running about. Wanted to hide, wanted to get away. Stayed in my room. Do that at home. Stayed in my room. Listened to it. Wanted to get away. Knew I had to get well to get out.'

'Bad experience, but you got well and got out.'

'Had to get away from it all, gave me the creeps. Not for me. Can't go back there. Had to get away.'

'Getting away sounds really important.' Charlotte left it open, simply empathising with the 'getting away'.

'Yeah.' Ali knew he did that a lot. But he needed to. Nothing wrong in that. Been like it for years. If he didn't like something he'd get away from it, find some way, either leave or, well, just hide inside himself.

Charlotte thought about whether she should say anything further. She simply repeated ' "getting away", so important for you'.

Ali nodded slowly. There were voices in his head, shouting at him. They'd been with him for a long while now. He didn't always hear them, but sometimes he did. They were always the same, calling him names, laughing at him. How he hated it. How he had hated them. But at the time, he'd just hated himself. Just wanted to get away. But he didn't want to talk about that. He pushed it away and brought himself back into the present.

'So, talking of getting away, is it time to go?'

'Well, I usually see people for 50 minutes, Ali. Time's not up yet, but if you want to go, that's fine by me. Can we just discuss whether you want to come back again, maybe talk some more about things? No pressure, up to you. I really mean that.'

Ali had promised Desmond, and his mum, that he'd give the counselling a go. He wasn't convinced. But he wasn't going to debate it now. 'Yeah, OK. Might as well.'

They agreed a time for the following week. 'Wish I could relax.' Ali was still very much on edge as he sat in the chair, his jaw tight, his body not really settling at all.

'How about trying a short relaxation exercise, it can help.' Charlotte was skilled in offering this and it was something that she knew many of her more anxious clients appreciated. She didn't know if it would help Ali, but it felt reasonable to offer it.

Of course, this could be viewed as being something outside of a person-centred way of working. The counsellor is introducing an idea from her frame of reference. Although it is being introduced because she is mindful of Ali's struggle to look relaxed in the session. Is it a reasonable idea to offer? How does it fit with the non-directive nature of person-centred working? Does it? There is an assumption that the client wants to be relaxed. Maybe part of him does, maybe not. But will it disturb the therapeutic process, or can it add to it?

'How d'you mean?'

'Well, I talk you into being relaxed just for a few minutes. Maybe a way to round off the session today.'

Ali pouted slightly but nodded. 'Yeah, OK, I'll give it a go.'

'OK, so, just sit back in the chair and if you want to, close your eyes.' Ali wasn't sure about closing his eyes, but he decided to do so.

'Now take a slow, deep breath, hold it a moment, and gently let it out, and as you do so, imagine your shoulders dropping slightly.'

Ali felt himself drop his shoulders. He hadn't realised quite how tight they had been feeling. Charlotte was speaking again.

'Now, take another slow, deep breath, hold it again, and let it out, and let those shoulders drop a little more.'

They did drop a little more.

'Keep breathing slowly and steadily.'

Ali continued to breathe slowly and steadily.

'Think of the number one, and just imagine yourself saying "one" as you breath out slowly.'

'O-n-e.' Ali breathed in again.

'Now t-w-o.'

'T-w-o.' Ali felt his shoulders drop a little more and his head felt heavy on the back of his neck.

'T-h-r-e-e.'

Ali was breathing in, and slowly he breathed out, imagining saying the word 't-h-r-e-e' as he did so.

'Feel the heaviness of your body. Just let yourself sit back into the chair, relax into it.'

Ali relaxed into it. Charlotte noted that the body movements had stopped and his face didn't look so drawn and tight.

'F-o-u-r.'

Ali repeated it on his next out breath.

'F-i-v-e.'

'F-i-v-e.' Ali began to feel a bit spaced out in his head, particularly behind his eyes, Almost a little bit floaty. It was nice.

'S-i-x.'

Ali heard Charlotte's voice, it seemed a little bit distant now. In fact, Charlotte had dropped her voice a little.

'S-i-x,' he repeated back to himself, silently feeling himself breathe the number out.

'S-e-v-e-n.'

'S-e-v-e-n.' Ali felt heavier and yet lighter, both at the same time. But he wasn't thinking about what he was experiencing, it was how it was.

'Think of a blue sky, bright blue sky on a still, warm day.'

Ali was there.

'As you breathe in, imagine breathing in that blue sky, breathing blue into your body, slowly, gently.'

Ali breathed the blue into his body. He could hear Charlotte's gentle voice. 'Blue in your nose, and filling your head, down your throat and into your lungs. Across your shoulders and down your arms to your hands.' Charlotte paused before continuing. 'Down your back and into your belly.' Another pause. 'Down your legs, your thighs, knees, calves, ankles, into your feet and out through your toes.'

Ali was calm and relaxed. He just sat there without thinking about sitting. He breathed without thinking about breathing. He relaxed without thinking of relaxing.

Charlotte didn't leave him for long, she only wanted to give him a sense of how he could be relaxed. She wanted him to have time to reorientate himself before leaving. 'Still breathing slowly, imagine the blue light draining down and taking with it all the tension in your body, like someone has taken a plug out in your feet and all the blue flows down, down into the earth, taking all the tension with it.'

Ali imagined the colour like a liquid draining away. As the blue level dropped he thought of his own colour once again, his brown skin emerging in his mind as the blue colour flowed down and out.

'Be aware of your breathing. Take a slightly deeper breath and be aware of the sensation of the chair against your body.' Charlotte could hear a bird calling outside in the tree. 'Listen to the bird.' A brief pause. 'Sense the taste in your mouth and any smells in the air.'

Ali's mouth didn't taste too good. The air felt warm.

'And in your own time, open your eyes, maybe stretch, maybe smile. Gently move your body.'

Ali began to stretch before opening his eyes. He opened them and blinked, the light felt strong in the room. He squinted and promptly felt a yawn coming on.

'Wow. How did you do that?' He was still stretching.

'How do you feel?'

'Good. Yeah, hey, that was good. How long was it, felt ages.'

'Just a few minutes. Do you feel different?'

'Yeah. Geeze, I feel, well, relaxed, really slowed down.' He stretched again, his back felt a little tight. It triggered another yawn. 'Can we do that again next week?'

'Sure. It's very simple.'

'Yeah. I feel good. That really took me to another place, you know? The sky just filled me up. It just floated into me. Wow.'

'OK, well, time's now up. Take your time as you go. You may feel a little unsteady. When you stand up, stamp your feet a little, ground yourself, yeah, get back in touch with the earth well, the carpet anyway!' Charlotte smiled.

Ali smiled back. He felt good. He was standing now and stamping on the carpet.

'See you next week. That was really great.'

Ali left feeling so different. It gradually faded, but it had made a deep impression on him. He didn't know he could feel like that, not without dope inside him. It wasn't the same, of course, but it was good. He liked the blue. Yeah, it felt good.

Charlotte smiled as she returned to her seat having shown Ali out. So few young people in her experience had really experienced a proper relaxation visualisation. It was simple really, she had done it many times and had learned to speak in a soft voice, and to get the timing right. She was always careful to watch the client's breathing and match her speed to their rhythm. She wrote up her notes.

Counselling session 2: Tuesday 12th May – client does not attend, letter sent to him

Charlotte looked at the clock again; Ali was now ten minutes late. She had felt sure he would attend after the experience of the last session. He had seemed so affected by the relaxation at the end. But time was passing and, well, there was nothing she could do but wait.

She sat quietly and thought about Ali. She was in the habit of doing this when a client did not attend or was late, and she wasn't sure whether they were coming. She believed that it was important for her to, in effect, still give her client time. She wouldn't sit for the whole 50 minutes, but she would make a point of just holding her client in her awareness and allow herself to feel positive regard towards him, or her. She smiled as she remembered Ali's reaction to the relaxation, but she could also see his very tight and angular expression previously in the session, his constant movement which, in a way, seemed almost as though he was constantly distracting himself. That was her meaning, quite what it meant for Ali she did not know.

After a further ten minutes she felt that she needed to make herself a drink and perhaps attend to something else. She hadn't lost hope of his arriving. It did happen. People getting delayed by transport problems, and not being able to make contact. So she maintained a state of mind that was expectant of Ali arriving whilst she went and made herself a cup of tea.

As she sat down with her drink she decided to write a letter to Ali, offering him another appointment. She wanted to express her sense of how their first session had been, and hoped to encourage him to come back, if that was what he wanted. She didn't send the standard form letter, she didn't believe they were appropriate. She knew her way took more time, but she wanted to be able to say something relevant to the client and to the contact they had already had.

Dear Ali,

I am sorry not to see you today. I hope you are not unwell. I guess you have a good reason for not coming.

I was so struck from our first counselling session how you responded to the relaxation. It seemed to have made a deep impression on you.

I can offer you another appointment for next week, Tuesday 19th May at 3.30 pm. I hope this will be convenient. If you do not expect to be able to attend, for any reason, can you give me a call and let me know?

I hope to see you next week.

With all good wishes,

Charlotte Walters

The wording of letters to clients who do not attend an appointment is important. The letter is still boundaried within the therapeutic alliance and therefore should reflect the attitudes and values of the person-centred approach: empathic, warm acceptance, congruence.

Summary

Ali is withdrawn in the first session, doesn't really want to say very much. He isn't sure that he wants to come back for another session but Charlotte invites him to experience a relaxation visualisation, which he does. It makes a powerful impression on him and Ali leaves feeling good and wanting to come back for more the next week. Ali does not arrive for the second session and there is no communication from him. Charlotte writes to him, hoping he is OK, acknowledging that he has probably not attended for a good reason, hoping to see him the following week and asking him to make contact if he does not expect to attend.

Points for discussion

- Assess counselling session 1. Would you have responded differently to Charlotte? How person-centred did you feel Charlotte was in the session?
- What were the key elements in that first session? What made the greatest impression on you, and why?
- What is your reaction to the relaxation? Did it seem appropriate?
- Why do you think Ali may not have attended, assuming he is well and would have been able to get to his appointment?
- How differently might you have worded the letter to Ali, and why?
- Would you inform anyone in the team that Ali has not attended? Justify your decision.
- If you were Charlotte, what issues would you take to supervision from this session?
- Write your own notes for session 1.

CHAPTER 7

A few weeks have passed. Ali did come the following week and has since attended the counselling sessions inconsistently. He has also missed some keyworking sessions. However, the service has stayed with him, seeking to maintain contact and to offer further counselling appointments and keyworking sessions. It has been a tough time for Ali. He has been compliant to the treatement and has kept to the medication much of the time, but there have also been occasions when he has given up with it and gone back to using cannabis. Each time it has been a reaction to a build-up inside himself, of feeling fragmented, edgy, unable to stop thoughts running in his head. It has made him depressed as well, his mood has swung but he has not had a recurrence of the experience that he had prior to going into hospital.

As the counselling sessions have continued, albeit sporadically, the relationship with Charlotte has deepened, although it has been a gradual process. Ali has not been consistent, at times it has seemed to Charlotte as though he presents different faces at different times, moving between them. This has been touched on but not in any great depth. When he has attended Ali has been more concerned with his present than with his past. Charlotte remains unaware of Ali's childhood, which he has chosen not to talk about. She has accepted this. She realises that at the moment the most intense experiencing for Ali is what is happening for him in the present. If you like, that's where the action is. She does not know if he will wish to explore beyond that, or, indeed, whether his own inner process will require this of him, or urge material from the past into sharper awareness and, perhaps, into the content of the counselling sessions.

Desmond has sought to motivate Ali to make changes to his lifestyle and he has made some progress. Ali does get out more and he has been thinking about a job again, though for now he remains signed off by his GP. He has helped out at a local charity shop and that has helped him to socialise a little. It is now session 7 with Charlotte.

Counselling session 7: Tuesday 16th June – the client reveals something of his childhood and identifies 'parts' of himself

'So, what do you want to focus on today, Ali?'

'The thoughts are racing around again and I'm feeling like I want to run away, but I can't, I can't run away from my own head. I ran away in the past, you know, on a number of occasions.'

Charlotte nodded. 'So running away is not new to you, you've done it before?'

'Literally. Used to just take off if things were too much. Ended up in Wales once, with no money. Mum and Dad had to come and collect me. They were pissed off, Dad in particular. Mum seemed OK, more worried and glad to see me safe.'

'All the way to Wales. Pissed your dad off, but your mum was glad you were safe.'

'Yeah.' He took a deep breath and sighed. 'Sometimes you have to get away.'

'Mhmm, gets all too much, I guess, and away you go.'

The counsellor has not directed the client to their feelings about running away, or how it affected him. Rather she has stayed with the client. By so doing she has not directed the client and therefore stayed in keeping with the theory of person-centred working.

'Part of me has always done that, wanted to run away. Goes back a long way.'

'So you mean you feel you've been running away for a long while?'

Another deep sigh. 'Yeah. Don't talk about it much.'

'Not easy?' Charlotte sought to empathise with the sense she was picking up from Ali that it was not easy to talk about this.

Ali shook his head. 'No, but it's what I do, and I know I'm doing it here. When I don't come, it's like playing truant – did that a lot as well. If I don't like something I go away. Get away, anywhere, just get away.'

'And that's what you've been doing, what, when you haven't come to the counselling sessions?'

Ali nodded. 'Yeah. And I don't know why. It's been really good and the relaxations you've done at the end of the sessions have really felt great. And I've learned to focus on them myself as well. Sometimes not too successfully, but at times it has made a difference.'

'I'm pleased. And yet you also need to ...' Charlotte almost said run away but stopped herself as she realised that Ali had only been talking of getting away, or had he? No, he'd said run away as well. She expressed her thoughts. 'I was going to say "run away" but thought you'd only said "get away", then realised you had said "run away".'

'Well, guess it was both really.'
'Both?'
'Yeah, and for a long time.'
'Running away and getting away, and for a long time.'
Ali nodded. He somehow felt it was right to be talking like this. He couldn't explain why, there was no reason why it should be any different this week, but it felt like he wanted to talk about different things, he felt an urge to talk more about his past. And even though it felt timely he also felt very uneasy as well. He put it down to talking about parts of his life that, well, were uncomfortable, and things he didn't generally talk about much – if ever.

Maybe the client was ready to talk before arriving for this session, maybe the way that Charlotte has stayed with him and not pushed him into his feelings has helped him to experience this sense of 'rightness' about what he was talking about. Yes, he is uneasy, it is an uncomfortable area, but he has perhaps been put at ease as well in some way by the counsellor's empathic responses and acceptance of what he has been saying.

There will be times when clients talk about areas of their life and experience that they have not previously shared with anyone. It takes time for trust to build, although there can also be occasions when the issues are so pressing that the client will talk throughout the first session, as though everything has been waiting until someone simply listened. However, in this case, it seems likely that Charlotte has earned Ali's trust and as a result the relationship moves on as an important part of his past is made visible.

'Goes right back to school.'
'What age?'
'Six, seven, something like that. Around the time my brother was born.'
'That seems a significant fact in all of this.'
'Well, meant Mum seemed to have less time for me. I can understand it now, but at the time, well, felt very much on my own.' Ali could feel his discomfort rising as he spoke. He could feel an urge to go quiet, say nothing more.
'Mhmm, on your own and no one to turn to?' Charlotte empathised with the experience rather than the factual description.
'Yeah.' He swallowed. The memory of the voices was re-emerging in his head. The taunts. The being talked about. Not having any friends, feeling very alone. He found himself sinking into his past, and into feeling quite low. He could also feel himself wanting to withdraw from Charlotte. He didn't want to talk about it, and he didn't want to feel about it either, or think about it. He closed his eyes, taking a deep breath. 'Yeah, bad times, but it was the past and I've got to get a grip on the present.'
'Yeah, the present's important to you; put the past behind you and get a grip on the present, yeah?'

The counsellor empathises and does not try to hold the client on the past. Clearly something happened, and some counsellors would hold the client's focus there. However, the person-centred counsellor acknowledges the client's wish to convey his need to get a grip on the present. That is what the client is saying and is therefore what, at this time, he wants the counsellor to hear. She stays with him, allowing him to develop what he was saying in his own way, at his own time and at his own pace.

'Something like that. But, well, I find myself thinking about the past a lot at the moment. Can't seem to let go of it. Thoughts go around, images, memories, voices . . .'

Charlotte did not simply seek clarification of the voices, but empathised with the totality of what Ali had sought to communicate to her. 'Can't seem to let go of the thoughts, images, memories and voices.'

Ali shook his head. He was feeling more anxious, as though the closer he got to something the worse he felt. He could feel a definite queasiness now inside himself, almost as though he might want to be sick. He swallowed. He took a drink of water from the plastic cup on the table. The water felt cool and he appreciated it.

'And I guess that . . . , oh I don't know. Sometimes I get really stuck, just don't know what to say next. I just want to feel better, you know, stop the thoughts, stop it!' He raised his voice. 'Sorry, I get so frustrated with it sometimes, and that's when I feel like I've had enough, when I want to go, just go away somewhere, anywhere, but it doesn't make any difference. Well, I mean, it does, going somewhere feels good, I like the idea of heading off, not knowing where you are going until you get there. That sort of appeals.'

'Taking off, anywhere, not knowing where. There's something about that idea . . .'

'Sure is. Yeah. Crazy, huh? Running away?'

Charlotte shook her head. 'May seem crazy to you, but not to me. Sounds like you felt you had a real reason why you chose to do what you did.'

The counsellor reassures the client, introducing her perspective, but is this an appropriate response. A response of 'seems crazy to you, running away?' may have been enough, however, as we shall see, the actual response is therapeutically helpful.

Ali nodded and took another deep breath. That felt somehow good. He hadn't been judged, in fact, Charlotte had not made an issue of it.

'Yeah, I always had a reason – in my head. Mightn't have been very sensible, but at the time, well, I had to do it.'

'Yes, sounds really important. You had to do it.' Charlotte emphasised the 'had' as she spoke, which reflected the emphasis she sensed that Ali was putting on it.

'Yeah. So, that was how it was.' Ali went quiet. He was back thinking about his childhood, how he'd been picked on so much at school, the trouble being in an area where there were few coloured kids. Got a bit better later in secondary school, though he'd given up by then. But at primary school ... He wasn't aware of it but he was slowly shaking his head.

Charlotte noticed the movement. 'Makes you shake your head thinking about it?'

Verbal responses to body language can be very powerful. Bodily movements can be direct expressions of what is being experienced, and may not be subjected to the same screening that may be applied to the spoken word.

'Mhmm.' Ali took a deep breath. He felt a little spaced out, and he felt a need to talk. It was like his past needed to reveal itself. Somehow it just felt the right thing to do. 'It was tough as a kid, you know. Well, anyway,' his hesitation was because he realised that Charlotte wouldn't know, wouldn't have had his experience, 'I got picked on and bullied. Mainly verbal stuff, called me names and stuff. Couldn't do anything about it. Couldn't talk about it at home. Had to put up with it. Really got to me. I was small as a kid, you know, just really didn't know how to cope. I'd try to keep away from school, tummy ache, headaches, you name it, I had it. Guess I learned to escape. Spent a lot of time on my own. Played games with myself, spent a lot of time thinking about things, feeling bad. I'd kind of escape into my own fantasy world where I was the hero, yeah, I was the one that they all had to respect. But that was on the inside, it wasn't real, but it was what I did. And if it got too much, I ran away. Not far, not then, the long trips came later, but that was 'cos by then I'd got to hate school.'

'So you'd escape into yourself, into a kind of heroic fantasy world, but you'd also physically run away, get away from things.'

'Yeah. It was like that for a few years. Changed schools when I was 11, the next school wasn't so bad. I mean, there were more coloured kids there. But I wasn't really interested in school. I'd also grown a bit by then and, well, got a bit more respect.'

'Like the fantasy figure you mean?' The thought struck Charlotte strongly that it seemed like he had started to live out the idea he had put so much thought into.

A spontaneous comment. Could be highly therapeutic, but in a sense it is making a connection for the client which he might have been better making for himself.

'Suppose so, hadn't thought of it like that. Yeah, well, I did get respect. Well, I'd got stronger and had a bit of a reputation. Wasn't vicious or anything, but, well, I'd do what I needed to do, though, kind of used to lose it a bit. That was how it was. Just went over the top I suppose.'

'Mhmm, so things would get out of control for you, do crazy things, go over the top?'

'Do anything. Someone dared me to do something, I'd do it.' He shook his head, but smiled as he thought back to those times. 'Then I'd go through periods when I'd go quiet, feel all moody. In a way that was worse, I'd get pissed off about something and then, well, then I could get angry. But it was because I felt bad, didn't want people in my space, didn't want to be bothered. It put people off. They didn't know how I was going to be, I guess. And, well, it was happening at home as well and, well, I ended up seeing the psychiatrists, you know. Didn't make much difference, nothing changed. I started smoking joints. Made me feel easier, stopped me dwelling on things, stopped the voices in my head, well, not really voices, but I'd kind of talk to myself, but yeah, I suppose I did kind of get voices in my head.'

Charlotte nodded, pleased that Ali was now talking about these early life experiences. It was helping her to more fully understand what had happened for him and maybe how it might be contributing to his problems today. 'So, voices started around then, and mood swings.'

Ali nodded. 'Yeah. And started smoking joints. I felt easier, not better, easier. But, well, I also lost interest in school even more. It wasn't good, not really. The doctors didn't seem to know what to do. Didn't want to really say much other than don't do it. Well, that wasn't going to stop me. And so it went on like that. Smoked more, felt less interested in things, left school. Had a few jobs, nothing special. Liked the last one – working at a nursery, doing stuff with plants and trees. But I lost that. They cut back. Last in, first out I guess. Then, well, things began to get worse.'

'So after you lost that job things got worse – the more you smoked, you mean?'

'No, wasn't like that. I was OK, I mean, I was up and down a bit but I handled it OK. Mum was worried. She cares about me, you know, but she does fuss as well. That gets me down.'

'Your mum fussing gets you down.'

'She's OK though, really. Seem to be talking to her a bit more now. She seems to be trying to get her life together – beginning to get out more. That's good to see.'

Charlotte smiled. 'That seems really important to her, and to you.'

'Yeah, it is. But I've got to get my life together now. God I still want a joint, been over a week now since the last one. Not been easy, though. And I'm still taking the medication. Still don't like to, but, well, Desmond encourages me to persevere. I have felt better with it I guess. I sleep a bit better. I take it at night, but I still have bad days, still feel like shit sometimes.' He shook his head.

'So, generally feeling better but bad days as well?'

Ali nodded.

Although Charlotte had reflected back what Ali had said, she did not know what he meant. In order to be more empathic she invited him to expand. She didn't want to just use his words without really appreciating exactly what it was he was experiencing. 'Guess I'm wondering what you mean by bad.'

Does the counsellor need to know? In a sense, Charlotte's response is an example of conveying an interest in what the client is saying, wanting to know what it is that Ali experiences and is trying to describe. This has therapeutic value. At the same time, it is directing him specifically to the 'bad' and his comment about feeling better gets lost. She may not know what 'bad' means, but does she know what 'better' means either? Why pick only on 'bad'?

'I don't know. I kind of withdraw into myself, and, well, thoughts start racing in my head. They've done that for years. It isn't as bad most of the time. The cannabis used to help, although I think the thoughts got crazier, particularly before I ended up in hospital.'

'So crazy, racing thoughts, that's what you mean by bad, Ali?'

He nodded. It wasn't easy to talk about them. Made him feel uncomfortable. He knew they were crazy but at the time it all seemed so real. So real. And he could feel the thoughts were still close, it wouldn't take much for him to get caught up in them again. Sometimes he did, he wasn't sure why, though he generally felt like he was being spied on, as though people could hear him through the wall or, when it was really bad, listen to his thoughts. That really unsettled him. It wasn't the thought that he believed these things that unsettled him, though, not at the time, anyway. It was knowing they were listening, listening to what was in his head and he couldn't shut them out.

That was when he really wanted a joint, just to make it all a little easier. Now he was trying to go without and he knew the thoughts were always close. They'd started up a few times this past week. He'd managed to divert his attention – that was something Desmond had been helping him with. He was helping him to identify the thoughts early on, or the feelings just before they started up, so he could try and focus on something else. It sort of worked, some of the time, but it wasn't really making them go away. He'd have these conversations in his head, lose all track of time. It was so easy for him to just sit and lose himself. He broke his train of thought. 'Sorry, I drift off so easily.'

Charlotte was thinking back to the first session, how anxious Ali had seemed, how he kept moving in the chair. He wasn't doing that so much any more, seemed more settled. She wasn't sure why it had suddenly struck her. She decided to own it and make it visible.

'I think I drifted off as well, back to thinking about the first counselling session, how unsettled you seemed to be in the chair. You're not like that now. You seem calmer. I don't know if that's how it feels, but to me it is how you look.'

The comment made by the counsellor is genuine, authentic and transparent. As we shall see, the client acknowledges it but it does not disrupt his need to continue talking about his thoughts and the effect they have on him. Sometimes in counselling, the counsellor can make this kind of transparent statement without it seemingly having any value. But that doesn't mean it hasn't been helpful. Just because a client does not pick up on it doesn't mean that it has not had some therapeutic significance. Often in counselling the counsellor will never know the effect of some of the comments they make. Whilst it is important to consider each specific response to the client, there is also a need to think holistically and consider the tone of the dialogue, and what that conveys, and what meaning that may have for the client. Here, Ali is with someone who is prepared to own their own thoughts. Who can tell what meaning he may attribute to this and what he will take away from the experience?

'Guess so. I do still get agitated though. I'm not always like this. The thoughts leave me agitated. The stuff on TV does as well.'

'Particular things on TV make you more agitated?'

'All the anti-Muslim stuff. They say it isn't but it is, and I'm not surprised people want to fight back. I've done some reading in a magazine about it. I can understand why people blow themselves up to kill people – they're desperate, some of them. Maybe not all, but some are, I'm sure.' He shook his head. He was thinking of the Palestinians. 'Generation after generation living in some camp in Palestine, not able to move around freely, poverty, and no sense of having much power to make a life for yourself. Yeah, I can imagine myself being prepared to do that. Why not? If there's nothing likely to change, same shit day in, day out, why not? Make a noise. Get heard. Do some damage. No one listens to anything else.' He shook his head. 'And I know that actually I probably wouldn't, probably go and smoke a joint instead to cope.' Though he said the final sentence, he wasn't totally sure. He had a feeling that maybe, maybe, that crazy part of him could do that. But then again, he wasn't sure how crazy it really was, not for someone brought up in one of those camps.

'But you can understand and part of you thinks you understand why some people take action, another part that you'd just smoke to cope.'

'Yeah, not really coping, just another way of getting away from it all, I guess. You can't run away – that's what I'd want to do, get out, get away, but if you can't do that, well, you smoke a joint to get away, don't you?'

'That's how it feels for you?'

'Yeah. I get that in my head, part of me wanting to hide away from it all, but that other part wanting to run away, break out of it, maybe be dramatic as well. Like when I went to Wales on the train, that was a statement, that was me breaking out.'

'Powerful statement, huh?'

Ali nodded. 'And, well, I guess that part of me still wants to break free, a kind of me that wants to just run away, yeah, break away from it all, from myself.'

'A kind of break away, run away sense of yourself.'

'It's part of me. It's not all of me, but it's part of me.'

'Mhmm, so part of you wants to break away.'

'Yeah. Part of me doesn't want to follow the rules, doesn't want to do what it's told to do, or . . .' He smiled. 'Or come to appointments, yeah?'

Charlotte nodded. 'Yeah, or come to appointments.'

'It's like one of the voices, telling me to just, what the hell, go for it, get out, get away, do it. It's the part that I guess caused me to do the crazy stuff when I was younger.'

'Mhmm. The crazy part. And, you know, sometimes it can be helpful to think of ourselves in this way, to identify the parts that make up who we are.' Charlotte wasn't sure quite how to voice this, but she was so very conscious of how Ali was talking about this crazy part of himself, the part that wanted to break free, not conform. It seemed to be an opportunity to perhaps help Ali to think of himself in terms of different parts. She had already begun to wonder how the parts might be linked to the voices and the thoughts in his head. She wondered what the crazy part told him to do.

Ali was taking a deep breath. At times he felt like he wasn't so much in parts as in bits. Thoughts in his head, voices telling him what to do, what to think, what to feel. Not always clear voices, often just thoughts, but they could so easily get out of control. 'And thinking about this, well, I guess there are lots of parts of me.'

'Mhmm, lots of parts, lots of parts that make you who you are.'

Ali nodded. 'Wish I could just mould them all together.'

'What, make them into one?'

'Yeah, like clay, just squeeze them together so they're not different any more, stop them talking to each other.'

'That how it feels, the parts of you talk to each other and you'd like to mould them all together to stop them talking?'

The empathic response could have been sharper, 'You want to stop them talking to each other?'. That's what is being conveyed through the words. The squeezing together is a way of achieving this. That's the process. The empathy could have been for the purpose behind the process, the need to stop the parts talking.

Ali nodded again. 'Maybe I'd feel better then. Maybe I'd feel better.'

'Mhmm, mould them all together and feel better.'

Ali was now shaking his head. 'But how? How do I do that? How do I take all this stuff in my head and . . .'. He put his hands out and made to squeeze some invisible substance together between his hands, '. . . how do I get hold of them, in me, whatever, how do I do it?'

'Yeah, how? You really want to.' Charlotte reflected back what Ali had said but also empathised with his wanting to stop the chatter in his head by moulding all the parts together. She reflected his hand movements. 'Seems hard to know what to get hold of.' That was how it struck her as she sought to mould her own invisible ball of parts.

'Yeah, I kind of need to know what the parts are, what I need to get hold of.'

'Mhmm, what are the parts that exist in your head, that make up who you are.' She voiced the reflection as a statement, not wanting to convey to Ali that she was asking him to tell her. 'You need to know what they are before you can get hold of them, that how it is?'

Ali nodded. Somehow it felt good talking like this, although he wondered if it wasn't just some new craziness that would just kind of go nowhere. And yet somehow it did make sense.

'So how do I do it?'

'What, identify the parts?'

Ali nodded slowly. 'I need to find some way of doing it.'

'Some way to identify all the parts that make you who you are.'

'Well, for a start there's the crazy me, the "want to break free" me. That's one.'

'Mhmm, OK, that's the first one.' Charlotte didn't say any more. She wanted Ali to gain his own insight and, importantly, find his own words or names to describe the parts that he identified. If he was to own them then he needed to define them. She waited to see what next came to mind for Ali.

'There's the part of me that just wants to withdraw, hide away, lose myself.' He tightened his lips and nodded to himself. 'And I guess that part of me likes me to smoke.' He smiled, remembering how he had smoked to hide in the smoke, hide from everyone who was listening to him trying to read his thoughts. He pushed this last thought away, he didn't want to go there.

'Mhmm, withdraw, hideaway, lose yourself.'

'It's not the bit of me that wants to get away by running away, I mean literally, but it does encourage me to get away, but in a different way. That's weird.'

'So a part that wants to run away, and a part that wants to hide away? Is that what you mean?'

As a client engages in a process like this of seeking to identify the 'parts' of themselves, it is vital that the counsellor allows the client to use their own definitions. It is not for the counsellor to start naming the 'parts'; it is for the client to do this. It may take a while for a final name to emerge, and it may never do, the 'part' remaining defined by a particular set of thoughts, feelings and behaviours. The 'part' exists within the client, it contributes to making him who he is. Only the client can really know what it means to him or for him. However much a therapist might feel they have a wonderful name for the 'part', they should refrain from suggesting it. The client is defining themselves to themselves. It is a subtle and important process, and can be easily disrupted by the well-meaning therapist introducing a name

> from their own frame of reference, with their associated meanings. Let the client find their own name and thereby intimately encounter their own natures through the lens of their own insight and experience.

That made immediate sense to Ali. 'Yes, hide away and run away. Similar but different. I guess they're two more parts of me although they both want to get me away from something – usually what's going on for me, or what's happening to me.' His thoughts slid back to his past. He nodded as he recognised how they had their origins in his childhood experiences. He'd sort of known it but somehow now he really knew it. 'I guess they kind of developed a long time ago.'

'Feels like they've been around a long time?'

'They were how I coped with the shit at school. Weird. Still living them, being them, I don't know how to describe it. But yeah, I can still want to run away – like not coming to my appointments – and I can withdraw, often into my room, but into myself as well.' Time was passing and the session did not have long to go. Charlotte mentioned this.

'Yeah, but this is interesting. I need to think about this more. Maybe I need to write it down in some way?'

'Mhmm, sounds good, write it down, map out all the parts.'

Ali was nodding in response. 'Guess I could draw it.'

'How would you draw it?'

'Don't know.' Ali lapsed into silence. He really wasn't sure. 'Guess I should just write them down.'

'Mhmm, just write them any old way?'

Ali shrugged. 'Don't know. Don't know what you mean.'

Charlotte thought about it for a moment and decided to offer Ali an idea. She sensed he was a bit stuck and had an idea as to how to go about it. 'Why not draw what's called a spider diagram – you in the middle with lines going out to all the parts.'

Ali nodded. He felt hesitant, he wasn't sure that was right, but it seemed like a good idea. He'd try it anyway. 'Ye-es, OK, so, lines going out from me with all the different parts kind of surrounding me?'

'Something like that. It's just an idea, but maybe you'll find a better way, your own way.'

'Maybe. I'll give it a go and, what, bring it back next week?'

'Sure, if you'd like to. I'd be interested in what emerges for you.'

'OK.'

> Would it have been better for Ali to have been left to do it his own way? It is not the first time that Charlotte has tried to help him when he is feeling stuck, or when she feels he needs something from her. Some might suggest that young people need direction and a more focused problem-solving

approach. However, in the context of therapy from a person-centred perspective, the client of any age needs to be allowed the freedom to find their own way, the counsellor being their companion in the exploratory process.

The person-centred counsellor should experience a deeply held recognition of the existence of the actualising tendency and genuinely hold a feeling of trust that the person has inner resources than can enable them to resolve their difficulties where the necessary and sufficient conditions for constructive personality change are being offered. This goes to the very heart of person-centred working. Without this belief – it is more than a belief, perhaps a conviction is a better word – then the counsellor cannot genuinely claim to be person-centred or to embrace the person-centred approach as a theoretical system for their therapeutic practice. Of course, where a client asks for a different approach then this can be negotiated and agreed, but the person-centred counsellor would still want the direction to flow from the client.

The spider diagram is actually a good way of mapping out parts, but care should be taken to avoid directing the client as to where to put the parts or locate the voices. It needs to emerge from the client's experience of themselves. It has been a bit hurried in the session and may have needed more exploratory time, and for Ali to have a sense of his freedom to express himself as he wants to, rather than any sense of having to do it a particular way because that is what the counsellor has suggested.

The session drew to a close and Ali left, still thinking about the parts of himself. Yes, he thought, there's certainly 'breakout me'. He thought of the Thin Lizzy song, 'Jailbreak', the bit where Phil Lynott says 'Breakout' and then the guitar riffs that follow. It was buzzy, it had energy. He'd listen to it when he got home. Charlotte returned to the counselling room. She felt good about the session. Glad that things had moved to where they had, with Ali taking an interest in himself. She wasn't sure whether she should have suggested the spider diagram, but it had seemed OK at the time. He seemed stuck. But then again, maybe she should have empathised with that, or voiced her sense of his being stuck. That would probably have been better. But, well, she'd said what she'd said now. And he could still do it a different way. But she was uneasy with the thought that he might take her suggestion as the right way to do it and therefore discount any ideas that he might have himself. That wasn't what she wanted.

It is worth commenting again on the content and responses in this session. Person-centred working requires the counsellor to be sensitive to the need to enable the client to begin to develop a greater internal locus of evaluation and be less dependent on, or conditioned by, external suggestions. As the theory says, we learn in childhood to base our judgement as to what is right or wrong from what others say, how others react. But they may not be right. And even if they are right, it means we develop a tendency to go with what others say rather than develop our own process of judging and decision making based on our own analysis or feelings about something. It is about learning to trust ourselves. So, by making the suggestion Charlotte may have unwittingly undermined Ali finding his own way of mapping out the parts that he feels make him who he is, and have impacted negatively on the process of movement from an external to an internal locus of evaluation. Importantly, however, in the process leading up to this, as has been said, she has left him to name and describe the parts. That is crucial. A counsellor can fall into the trap of naming them based on what they sound like to him or her, but for there to be real ownership, for the client to really feel that they are engaging with and describing a part of themselves, they need to associate their own meanings with it, their own thoughts, feelings, behaviours and, if they choose to do so, their own name.

Counselling session 8: Tuesday 23rd June – psychotic event in the counselling session, 'parts' identified

Ali was a few minutes early, he hung around outside having a cigarette. The sun was shining. He felt on edge, bit more than usual. He was still taking his medication, but he was still finding things difficult. It had been a bad week at home. His father had had a go at him. He reacted and smashed a vase. He'd picked it up and his father had said, 'Don't you dare smash it. You're out of here if you do.' Ali hadn't hesitated, his response instantaneous. The vase was thrown down and he walked out, slamming the door behind him. His dad was furious. There was a huge row and his mother had come home in the middle of it and had to try and separate them. Things eventually calmed down. But it hadn't been easy all week since that incident.

He finished his cigarette and rang the bell. The receptionist saw him on the CCTV and, recognising him, pressed the button to let him in. She called Charlotte on the phone and she came out to find him. He followed her to the counselling room.

'So, where do you want to begin today?' She sensed immediately that Ali didn't seem very settled.

'Feeling pissed off. Dad had a go, I broke a vase and, well, he's been having a go ever since.'

Charlotte nodded, 'And that's made you feel pissed off.'

He moved in the chair. 'Yeah. Bastard. Always looking for an opportunity to have a go.'

'That's how it feels, like he's looking to have a go at any opportunity.'

'Yeah. But he deserved having that vase broken. Daring me to do it.'

'So he dared you to break it and, well, you did.'

Ali was staring down at the ground. He suddenly looked up, his eyes were staring more than usual. 'Yeah, and I'd do it again. Daring me to do something.'

Charlotte felt very strongly that there was now something very different about Ali. He'd been a lot of things in the sessions, but this was new to her. He looked kind of, well, sort of bewildered, perplexed, there was almost a wild-eyed look that flashed across his face as he had spoken, yet somehow the word 'crazy' came most strongly into her mind.

'Feels to me like it must drive you crazy.'

'Yeah,' Ali nodded.

An interesting empathic response, merging the emphasis on how the client was feeling with the way he is looking in the 'here and now' of the counselling session.

'And you feel this way, what, when someone dares you to do something?'

'Well, he shouldn't mess with me, you know, he shouldn't.'

Charlotte nodded, she wasn't going to reflect back what he had said, she felt her empathy was likely to sound a bit parrot-like. 'No, messing with you like that makes you feel crazy.'

Ali looked away, as suddenly as he had looked up moments before. 'Yeah, so, that's how it is.' He continued looking away, seemingly staring at something on the wall but there was nothing there, just the paint.

'Mhmm, that's how it is.' Charlotte felt her own tension. She was aware that her concentration had increased, but she was also aware that she was sitting further forward than she might usually do. She thought about relaxing back into the chair but wondered what that would communicate. So she maintained her posture and kept her focus on Ali, waiting for his next response.

'I need to go. I really need to get the fuck out of here.'

'Something makes you want to leave?'

'I don't want to sit here like this for an hour. Waste of time. Waste of fucking time.'

'So you need to go because it feels a waste of time being here, yeah?'

Ali could hear a voice in his head telling him 'Go on, get out, go home, go and break something. Show you're not scared of him. Go on. You know you want to do it. That black vase on the piano, you've always thought how ugly it is. Go on. Waste it. Show him you don't give a fuck.' Ali closed his eyes and his breathing became heavier. No, he didn't want to do what the voice was saying, well, actually he did, but he didn't as well. 'No.' He shook his head.

Charlotte noticed the body movements. 'No?'

Ali took a deep breath. He didn't want to say about the voice. It wasn't often there, but when he got mad about something it could sometimes start.

'Nothing.'

'Nothing?'

Ali shook his head. 'Go on, get the fuck out of here. What does she know. Get the fuck out of here. Go and do some damage.' The voice in his head was persistent.

'No, for fuck's sake.' Ali took his head in his hands and ran his fingers back through his hair. 'No.'

'What's happening in your head, Ali, can you tell me about it?' Charlotte spoke softly. She was genuine in her response. She could sense that something powerful was happening for Ali and she wanted to offer him the opportunity to talk about it.

Ali took a deep breath and made to speak, but closed his mouth, breathing out heavily through his nose. 'No, I . . . Oh fuck it.'

'What is it Ali? Take your time. I only want to understand what's happening for you.'

Ali had only really talked to Desmond about the voices he sometimes had in his head. Desmond had given him some ideas for controlling them. Often it worked. He could recognise the feelings before they began and would divert his focus, often doing something physical could make the difference. They came and went. He'd always controlled them in the past with the cannabis, at least, that was how he had experienced it, although he'd always felt no one had believed him, until now, anyway. Just now the voices seemed to be more frequent. He shook his head.

'Must be scary to experience what you're experiencing, Ali, maybe I can help?' Charlotte knew she wasn't being very empathic but she felt she was offering Ali her wish to understand and to help. She hoped that she was able to communicate her presence, and her sense of unconditional positive regard for him. She did not want to lose psychological contact with him, though she also recognised that he may well become so absorbed into his own world that she became invisible to him. She wanted to remind him of her being there for him, with him.

Ali had closed his eyes and was clearly concentrating. His body looked tight like a coiled spring as he sat there, not moving except for the occasional twitch, as though his muscles were going into spasm. His jaw was set firm. He knew he had to focus on something else, do something. He suddenly stood up, his fists clenched, and began banging his wrists together, faster and faster, until his arms ached and he could do it no more.

Charlotte recognised that the behaviour had to be for a reason. She didn't feel threatened by it. Although in a sense it was a violent act, she somehow felt an empathy for something that she sensed to be underlying the physical action. She remained calm, trying to feel her way into what Ali's world was like, and realising that in reality she couldn't. Parts of a passage from a paper by John Schlien came into her mind, 'the true nature of psychosis is a mystery . . . indescribable from the inside . . . incomprehensible from the outside . . .' (Schlien, 1961). She chose not to dwell on it, but it summed up the challenge of working with, and communicating meaning, where a psychotic episode was concerned.

'Let us recognise that the true nature of psychosis is a mystery. . . One of our problems, then, is how to deal with a subject consisting of experience which at its worst is indescribable from the inside and incomprehensible from the outside, and this without using words which are themselves confounding. 'Psychosis', for instance, has an authoritative, antiseptic sound, but its real sterility lies mainly in its lack of clear meaning. It simply replaces 'madness' – now a literary term, and 'insanity' – which represents a dated legal concept. Falling into pseudoscientific conventions of language will not help. At the present stage of knowledge the questions are well enough represented by asking simply: What does it mean to 'lose one's mind'? How can a 'lost mind' be recovered?' (Schlien, 1961)

She felt unsure what was happening but she wanted to trust whatever process was occurring. She was not sure how much psychological contact there was between them and she decided to make a 'pre-therapy response', seeking to make reflective contact through the actions that Ali was displaying.
'You hit your wrists together and you stop.'
Ali had not heard her. The voice was still there and it filled his head. 'Get the fuck out of here.' He stood still, he was not aware of anything. His eyes were glazed. He suddenly sat down.
'Ali sits down.' Charlotte again sought to reflect the movement in her response, no more and no less.
Ali continued to sit.
'I am sitting with Ali in the counselling room.'

The responses Charlotte is making are pre-therapy situational reflections. In these responses 'the therapist looks at the client's current situation, environment or milieu and reflects the client's related behaviour' (Prouty *et al.* 2002, p. 16).

A minute passed during which Ali heard the voices of the children in his head, screaming at him and taunting him. They would tie his wrists together and sometimes leave him tied against something, and he'd be frantically trying to release his wrists. But this memory was not clear to him, he just heard the voices.
Charlotte reflected Ali's continuing to sit. 'Ali is still sitting.'

This is a reiterative reflection, embodying 'the principal of re-contact' (Prouty *et al.* 2002, p. 16). Here the intention is to reflect a continuation of a particular behaviour, for instance, in order to attempt to make re-contact with the client.

Ali took a deep breath. He wanted the voices to go away. He screwed his eyes
up tight.

'Ali screws his eyes up tight.' Charlotte stayed with the body language and movement, it was all she had to respond to. She was unsure what was happening for
Ali, but she was not going to try and pull him out of his experience. She wanted
to trust his process. She knew she had to keep her reflections minimal, to seek
some level of psychological contact, however minimal.

The counsellor gives a facial reflection, 'the therapist looks at the client's
face and observes pre-expressive affect' (Prouty *et al.* 2002, p. 16). Prouty
indicates the importance of this type of reflection as being particularly
necessary 'with regressed clients because excessive tranquilisation, psychosocial isolation, or institutionalisation lead to an atrophy or defensive
numbing of affective expression' (Prouty, *et al.* 2002, p. 16).

'... have to. Noises. Voices. Aaaiiyaa.'

'... have to. Noises. Voices. Aaaiiyaa.' Charlotte reflected the words and the
sound, not knowing quite what Ali was experiencing, but she sought to gain
at least the possibility of some psychological contact with him.

'Many psychotic clients often function at sub-verbal level, expressing word
fragments, incomplete sentences, or isolated words ... the therapist listens
carefully and reflects the word, even if he does not understand its meaning'
(Prouty *et al.* 2002, pp. 16–17).

The voice returned telling him to 'shut the fuck up'. Ali got up and started the
same wrist-hitting movement he had done before.

'Ali hits his wrists together faster and faster.'

He heard Charlotte's voice. It seemed distant. It was telling him something, it was
telling him ... wrists, hits, faster. Wrists, hit faster. He was ... his wrists, faster
and faster, he was ..., his wrists, his wrists. He had to break free, had to break
free, had to, had to ... He felt himself becoming clearer, he could feel his wrists.
Ali stopped and dropped his hands. He opened his eyes and with one movement
sat straight back down again. He took a deep breath. He looked a bit bemused.
He blinked.

'You OK?'

He nodded. 'I think so.'

As mentioned earlier, pre-therapy is a way of seeking to establish some
degree of psychological contact with a client in order to engage with them
in psychotherapy. In this instance, the client has entered into a psychotic

state, and has moved what would have seemed to the counsellor to be out-side of psychological contact with her. She therefore employs pre-therapy reflections in order to maintain contact during the period of the psychotic episode. Her reflections seek to enable her to have contact with the client, and the client with her. And at the same time, connect the client to what he is saying or doing. The latter can help the client, in this situation, begin to regain his sense of body-awareness and his usual sense of self.

For further reading on the theme of application of pre-therapy when working with psychiatric patients with severe mental disturbance, readers are referred to: Van Werde (1998); Deleu and Van Werde (1998); and Pört-ner (2000).

To Charlotte, Ali seemed to be more present again. 'What happened?'

Ali hesitated. 'You don't want to tell her,' the voice in his head screamed at him. Did he want to tell her? He stayed silent for a short while. He took another deep breath. 'OK.' He breathed out. 'OK, I get voices in my head sometimes, telling me to do things. I've talked to Desmond about it and he's helping me to control them, because I used to smoke dope, but, well, I haven't got that and the med-ication helps some of the time but when I get wound up, well, they start up. And it just happened. And I lose it, like just now.'

'The voices are with you now?'

Ali nodded.

'Can you tell me what they are saying?'

'Telling me to shut up and get the fuck out of here. Telling me to stop talking to you. Telling me to go and break something, smash something.'

'Mhmm, so there's a voice in your head telling you to shut up, get the fuck out of here and go and smash something.' Charlotte stayed calm. She had worked with clients with this kind of experience before, although she acknowledged that everyone was different and that there was likely to be some meaning for Ali as to why the voices existed and said what they said. That, at least, was the premise from which she worked.

As a person-centred counsellor, Charlotte will take the view that what is happening for Ali is an expression of his own psychological processes and that what is occurring will have meaning to him. The content of what is being said may be seen as emerging from an aspect of himself. That part of him wants to keep him quiet, wants him to leave, wants him to break some-thing. This is likely to stem from past experience and the fact that the voice appears to Ali separate from himself – in other words, as though someone else is telling him what to do – would suggest that this 'part' within his self-structure was generated with an intensity at some point in his life such that it has a certain degree of separation from his normal awareness. The person-centred counsellor will want to hear this 'part', offering it the same core conditions that she would wish to offer Ali or any other client. By so doing she can help Ali relate more fully to this 'part' of himself in order to break down the separating barrier with the hope of integrating this 'part' more fully into his structure of self. It is not unreasonable for someone feeling under stress or threatened, or perhaps frustrated with themselves, to want to run away, or keep quiet, or want to smash something.

Ali nodded.

'And that's something that only the voice wants you to do?'

Ali thought about it. The voice was saying it and, yes, part of him did want to do what it said, but another part of him didn't. He wanted to stay and make sense of it all, but he felt. . . The voice was speaking again, telling him to get out, to get out now. He closed his eyes. It just left him hearing the voice more clearly so he opened them again. He wasn't going to leave. He somehow felt he could trust Charlotte. She didn't seem to be unduly anxious, she seemed quite steady. He shook his head and spoke. 'No, not just the voice, part of me wants to go as well.'

'So part of you wants to get away.'

'Doesn't feel like a part of me, feels, well, separate, it really does, I just hear it in my head. But it's not me, I don't think it's me.'

'OK, not part of you, but it speaks to you?'

Ali nodded.

It is unlikely that clients will immediately feel able to accept the voice, or voices, that they are hearing as parts of themselves, or as emanating from parts of themselves. This insight may emerge over time as the therapeutic process develops, as a greater continuity of awareness is established within the client between the various parts of themselves. However, for some people, the voices will always be perceived as external to their sense of self.

'But another part of you doesn't want to do what it says?'

Again Ali nodded. His jaw was set firm. 'Yeah, that does feel like me, the part that doesn't want to do what the voice says.' He nodded to himself. Yeah, he thought, that's how it is. 'I've got to face this, I'm not running from it, but I don't know, it feels fucking awful sitting here.'

'Must be really uncomfortable, feeling the battle inside yourself like this.'

Ali took a deep breath. 'Is it part of me speaking? I don't know. Just doesn't feel like it, feels outside of me, coming into my head, but then it's in my head as well.' He paused, staring ahead of him, then shaking his head. 'It's weird 'cos just now I kind of remembered for a moment how it was in the past, the bullying and stuff, getting picked on, being called names – being tied up. That was the worst. The names, well, I just wanted to run away, but they'd tie my wrists to something . . .' Ali felt a surge of emotion. He closed his eyes and swallowed hard. 'I'd want to smash something in my frustration, although usually I'd just hide away when they let me go.'

Charlotte could feel her heart going out to Ali, and she guessed her own pain would be visible on her face. 'So much frustration, tied up, called names, desperate to hide away.'

Ali stared ahead of him, nodding slightly. Something seemed to shift inside him. The voice he had been hearing, he could somehow hear it as an echo from the past, it did seem like a mix of the taunts and his own anger and frustration at wanting, but not being able, to get away. And yet it still didn't completely feel like it was him. But he knew in a somehow more knowing way that it did all go back to his past experiences at school. 'It all goes back to the past, doesn't it?'

Charlotte nodded. 'It clearly feels connected to the past for you.'

'Yeah, but I don't understand it. I mean, yeah, I had a hard time, but kids do, and, well, they don't all end up like me, seeing doctors and then, well, ending up like this, you know?'

'Mhmm, it's not easy to make sense of.'

'I wish I could, I really do. I hate feeling the way I do, I hate feeling like I'm, well, it's just a constant fight inside myself. But you don't seem particularly anxious. But it feels like I'm going mad and people treat me like I'm going mad. I mean, the psychiatrist kept telling me I needed medication to help me be normal. But I am normal. I just hear voices sometimes and they sometimes make me go crazy with the tension.'

Charlotte nodded and noted the rising anxiety in Ali's voice as he spoke.

'Yes, it can feel like you're going mad and some people think you are, but that's not really how you want to see it?'

'Am I mad? Am I, really?' Ali looked at her straight in the eyes. In that moment he needed to know. Something in him wanted desperately to know that he wasn't mad.

Charlotte knew she could not hesitate but had to answer immediately. Hesitation could be misinterpreted as meaning she was having to think about what she said. Ali wanted to know, and know now.

'No. I think you have some problems and I want to help you find ways of resolving them. I think it's good that you have had a difficult experience here, now, and have come out of it, and without using cannabis or anything else to cope, or even the exercises you've been using. You've contained it.'

An important acknowledgement that Ali has managed the episode himself and kept it contained. Of course, the risk is that the client will not hear this because his own experience may have felt very different. Perhaps the counsellor could have qualified her comment through ownership, 'it seems to me that you have contained it'.

Ali nodded, that was unusual. 'And you didn't run away.'

Charlotte smiled, 'No, no, I didn't.'

'I think it frightens people.'

'It is frightening to see, but, well, I wanted to be with you and allow you to be as you needed to be.'

'You make it sound kind of OK.'

'People have all kinds of experiences, some quite extreme.'

'But you don't think I'm mad?'

Charlotte shook her head, 'No, no I don't think you're mad. Is that what you think, though?' Charlotte wanted to put the focus back on Ali's thoughts about himself. She knew that by responding directly to his question she was not allowing his internal locus of evaluation to be strengthened; quite the opposite – unless what she had said was also what he thought and so it might help him to feel he could trust his own thinking a little more.

'Sometimes. I guess I know I'm not, but sometimes...' Ali didn't finish the sentence.

Charlotte nodded and smiled slightly. 'Yes, sometimes it must feel like that even though you know you're not.'

'I want to be normal, I really do. Sometimes I think I don't know what normal is.'

'Being normal's really important for you but, as you say, what does it mean?'

'Not having voices in my head telling me to do things. But it's not just that. In a way I've really done a lot to control that. Desmond's helped me a lot, it's just feeling on edge so much of the time, and feeling, I don't know, I just don't feel together, somehow. It's hard to explain.'

Charlotte nodded and sought to empathise whilst also clarifying her understanding. 'So it's like you don't feel "together", but it is hard to explain exactly what you mean by this.'

'It's like I feel pulled about, like, well, you talk about part of me telling me to do things. I don't know if there are lots of parts of me, the voices, I don't know. But if there are – bit like we talked about last week – bits of me wanting to act different or be different ... I don't know. I get confused. I get lost in it all.' His expression looked really pained and Charlotte's heart went out to him. She knew she had no idea whether what he was experiencing was simply a reaction to his early life experiences, or whether he had developed a problem linked in some way to a chemical imbalance perhaps, or that the cannabis use had itself triggered something or at least exacerbated what was already happening for Ali. But not only did she not know; it wasn't important for her as a person-centred counsellor to know.

The counsellor's role is to form a therapeutic relationship with the client; to enable him to experience a trusting relationship formed from the presence of empathy, congruence and unconditional positive regard. If this can be achieved then Charlotte trusts that Ali's own actualising tendency would be freer to help him move towards a more satisfying sense of self and if the 'parts' could be drawn back together and owned, then he could move on as a much more 'together' person, to use his own words.

'Sounds like a lot to get lost in, Ali.'

'Does my head in. Makes me go crazy. I mean, not mad crazy, but, you know ...'

Charlotte nodded, 'Yes, you lose the plot, yeah?'

Ali nodded. 'Things just wind me up, Dad winds me up. Sometimes I want to stand up to him, other times I want to just hide away.'

'Two different responses from within you.'

'Yeah. Sometimes I just react one way, and sometimes another. This week he just wound me up.'

'Mhmm, and I'm wondering what it was that wound you up?'

'The way he has a go, and then daring me to break that vase. No one dares me to do anything, well, that's how it's been.'

'And that goes back to school experiences, yes, what you were saying about getting some kind of credibility?'

'Yeah, and I needed it.' He paused. 'But what about the voice. You're right, it does feel like part of me. I suppose I'd not really thought about it like that much. I kind of thought it was something wrong with me, I mean, like, I don't know, everyone kept blaming it on the pot, but I knew it wasn't that. That helps. It keeps me settled, you know?'

Charlotte knew only insofar as she heard what Ali was saying. 'I hear you, Ali, for you the cannabis helped, but it's being blamed for how you are sometimes.'

Ali rubbed his forehead quite intensely. He felt tired, his eyes were suddenly gritty and he yawned.

'Last week, we talked about me drawing the parts of me? I didn't do it. I sort of intended to but it didn't happen and then, well, you know what happened and I never felt like doing it much after that. But I do want to do that.'

'OK, is that something you want to do now?' Charlotte glanced over to the clock, there was still plenty of time.

'Yes, I tried thinking about it. I liked the idea of part of me wanting to break out, made me think of the Thin Lizzy song, "Jailbreak". Know that one?'

Charlotte nodded.

' "Tonight there's gonna be a jailbreak", yeah?'

'Mhmm.'

'Well that's part of me, I kind of called it "jailbreak" 'cos that's how it felt when I thought about it, needing to break out.'

'So, "jailbreak" is the part of you that wants to break out, break away, is that the same as wanting to run away?'

'Sort of.'

Charlotte nodded. 'Mhmm.'

'And that's also me wanting to get away from stuff in the past, yeah, going off on journeys, getting out, getting away.'

'Sounds like a really dynamic part of you, and maybe a really powerful part.' Charlotte was responding to the strength in Ali's voice as he talked about this part of himself. 'Sounds good to hear you talking with that power.'

Ali was slightly taken aback by the comment. It sounded good, but surprising as well. 'Yeah, well.' He suddenly felt embarrassed.

Charlotte noticed a darkening flush on his face. 'Can be difficult sometimes to hear a positive response like that?' She wasn't intent on making her comment a question, although it seemed to come out that way.

'Don't get many positive things said about me. But you think power's good?'

'Can be, guess it's what you do with it and how you feel about that.'

'Yeah, well, breaking out feels good. I need more of that.'

Charlotte nodded and thought to herself, OK, maybe this part is where his actualising tendency is going to focus if he is to break out and away from his cannabis use.

'You need more of that sense of breaking out, like you need to feel that "jailbreak" a bit more, yeah?'

'Yeah. That would be good.' He nodded to himself. The song was going through his head, 'Tonight there's gonna be trouble'. 'Yeah.' He gazed into space. He wasn't thinking anything in particular, simply sitting staring. He could hear the guitar riff in his head, it felt powerful. He needed that kind of power.

Charlotte watched him as she sat opposite. He seemed miles away and yet very present. She didn't feel that this was a silence in which he had disappeared, no that was the wrong word, engaged with some deep part of himself that might be slightly detached from his usual reality. She had seen that happen with clients, how they engage with a part of themselves that has some degree of dissociation. But this wasn't one of those moments, as far as Charlotte was concerned. She respected the silence and waited.

'Good song, good guitar sound, makes me feel strong thinking about it.'

'Sounds like that part of you could be strengthened by it?'

'Maybe not just that part, you know. It's weird, you know, thinking like this. I mean, I left last week feeling really good about thinking about all these different parts of me. Something really good about it. I was kind of curious and, yeah, it felt right even though it felt weird.'

'Mhmm, right but weird.'

'So, yeah. Can I write this down? You said last week something about putting myself at the centre and drawing the different parts. I thought about that, but I'm not sure I want to do it like that. Have you anything I can draw on?'

'Sure.' Charlotte found a sheet of A4 paper and a pencil. 'There you go.'

'I kind of think I'm like this.' He drew a kind of pinman but with a large head. 'And it's all in here, you know? So,' he drew a circle inside the head, 'this is "jailbreak", yeah.'

'Mhmm, OK. So "jailbreak"'s in your head?'

'And that's where I think all of the parts of me should be, you know?' He frowned. Did he mean that? He had said before that the voice hadn't seemed to be him, or a part of him, and yet . . . Now he wasn't so sure, but he didn't know why.

'OK, so all the other parts of you are in there as well.' Charlotte had not picked up on Ali's frown, she was looking at the paper.

An opportunity missed to acknowledge the frown, and possibly as a result the client might have explored his awareness that his thinking was changing

> about the voice in his head. Observing the client's reactions to their process of expressing themselves on paper is as important as what they are drawing or writing. The counsellor needs to endeavour to be empathically responsive to all that the client is communicating.

Ali drew another circle. 'That's the bit of me that wants to hide away, that wants to disappear when things are bad.' He sat silently for a moment, nodding as he looked at the circle with the words 'hide away' written in it. 'That's where I go. That's the place I hide in, I guess.' He stopped and thought about it. 'I guess that needs to be a small circle so I can feel small 'cos that's how it feels' (Ali's pinman drawing, p. 152).

'Mhmm, so when you disappear it feels like you go small?'

Ali nodded. 'That's the bit of me that just freezes and wants to hide when something awful happens. That's school stuff, when I couldn't fight back. I just froze and wanted to be invisible. Wanted to hide inside myself.'

Charlotte remembered something that she thought Ali had said previously, but she wasn't sure. Was it her imagination, or had he said something about smoking the cannabis to hide in the smoke? She wasn't sure. Should she say anything? It felt like she'd heard him say it. She decided to trust the process that had brought it into her mind.

'You said something previously, I think, some while back, about smoking cannabis to hide in the smoke, is that right, or am I imagining it?'

> Why has Charlotte said this? It has diverted Ali's focus. She has lost her empathy and is unaware that it has happened, so full of her own thoughts. Though the memory of what Ali had said may be right, why introduce it now? A response along the lines of, 'so desperate to hide away inside yourself . . .' would have sufficed and been a genuinely empathic response. It is possible that there is something in Charlotte that is blocking her from engaging with this area of Ali's experience. It should be a supervision issue, but Charlotte has not noticed it.

'Yeah, That's right that's how it is, well, was, you know?'

'Mhmm.'

Ali was thinking about what Charlotte had said. It was bringing back some sweet memories, that lovely sense of how it could be, a kind of mellow brightness. He breathed deeply, seemingly trying to breathe the memory back into his body. He could feel the urge to smoke a joint. That sense of wanting to drift into that other world, that other space inside himself. Hide away, and yet become himself as well. Drift into that place where everything seemed OK. He was smiling.

'Good memory, huh?' Charlotte was smiling as she spoke, guessing what was probably going on for Ali.

He nodded. 'Yeah.' He snorted, 'Don't think I'll really stop, just need to get myself together and smoke the odd joint just to keep the experience alive. Not something you can deny yourself once you've experienced it, you know?'

Actually, Charlotte did know. She'd smoked a few joints in her time, but didn't want to get into a sharing of drug-taking experience with him. 'Hard to imagine not engaging with that experience again.'

'Yeah. But you know, the relaxation we did, that first session, I know we've done a couple since, but that one really did feel good. It really did. I'd like to do that again.'

'Sure. Now?'

Ali looked down at the piece of paper he had begun drawing the image of himself on.

'No, let's get this finished. I got as far as "hide away", yeah, that's a good name for it, "hide away".' He wrote it in the bubble in his head. 'OK, so, that's "jailbreak" and "hide away". I like it. That does feel like how it is, looking at this, two bubbles in my head, two worlds, both places to escape into.' He paused for a moment. 'Yeah, both give me a place to get away to, but there's . . . , no, it needs to be different, doesn't feel right.'

'Mhmm, something doesn't feel right about what you've drawn or written?'

' "Jailbreak", I don't know, no, both of, they both kind of take me out of my head as well as into it. That's weird. Know what I mean?'

'Both ways of getting away from what you're experiencing?'

'Yeah, but they don't really take me away from myself, I'm still in my own head, aren't I, however different it might feel? So maybe it's OK like that.'

'You're still in your head even though it's like a movement away from yourself?'

Ali nodded. 'But "jailbreak" 's got power, "hide away" hasn't. "Hide away" 's escaping, running. "Jailbreak" 's sort of like that, but it's positive. Like when I went off as a child, I'd just go, get away, literally. I didn't know where I was going but it was somehow positive. Yeah, more positive. "Hide away" 's negative.'

'So "jailbreak" is positive, "hide away" is negative?'

'Still not sure that's right. Anyway, doesn't matter. That's how it is. So, "jailbreak" 's the voice in my head.' He nodded. 'Seems somehow less scary now that I can think of it like this. It's part of me, and I don't have to be scared of it, and I don't have to listen to it, do I?'

Charlotte was shaking her head. 'You don't have to, it's up to you, it's part of you.'

'Yeah.' Ali felt strangely calm, as though he had found some temporary peace. 'And it all goes back to the crap at school, and feeling hopeless and helpless and everything.'

Charlotte nodded. She was struck by just how well Ali was working with this way of looking at himself. It seemed to have particular meaning for him, helping him to make sense of who and how he is. She wasn't so naïve as to believe that it was going to take the voices away, but if it helped him to gain some understanding and control, she felt sure it would help.

Time was passing and the session was coming to an end. 'So, is this helping, Ali?'
He nodded. 'It's really making me think a bit, and that's no bad thing. But I feel tired, you know. And I think it's important that I'm seeing Desmond as well. You're both really different, but it feels good to be able to just talk like I do here, and, yeah, "jailbreak" and "hide away", yeah, they're certainly parts of me.'

'Well, something to think about and, when you're ready, we can maybe take it further. But only when you're ready.'

He nodded. The session closed and Ali decided he wanted to leave what he had drawn with Charlotte, and come back to it the next session.

As he left, Charlotte pondered on the possible reasoning for his decision. Did he not feel ready to take it out from the counselling space? Was that symbolic of something? Or was it that he didn't want to lose it or get it crumpled in his pocket? She didn't know, and realised she didn't need to know. She accepted his need to make his decision and that was all that mattered. 'Jailbreak' and 'hide away'; she smiled as she thought about the concepts. And both of them will have their own associated thoughts, feeling, behaviours. And all going back to being bullied and picked on because of his colour at school. She shook her head. How little we appreciate the damage that can be done in childhood. It may not always seem extreme, but the structure of self is being affected and then, well, later in life the person has to contend with fragmentation or divisions within their psyche. And then there's the growing use of substances amongst young people. How is that affecting development and particularly when these kind of damaging processes are already under way? She took a deep breath, feeling a little bit of despair looking at a society that didn't really seem willing to cater for the need amongst young people to deal with drug-related issues and problems related to emotional and psychological development.

Charlotte didn't like the emphasis that was always placed on mental health. It was generally far more accurate to think in terms of emotional and psychological processes. Mental was mind and thinking. That was not where most people's problems had their roots. Emotional disturbance, inability to contain feelings, lack of ability to feel, desensitisation to repeated exposure to ridicule or bullying, or oversensitivity, so many variations could occur as a result of traumatic experience. And there was Ali. The word 'persecuted' came to mind. Persecuted because of his racial and perhaps cultural, maybe even religious, differences. Made to feel a particular way about himself as a result. Made to have to try and hide away, and then in times of desperation needing to run, break out of the jail that was being constructed within his structure of self. She sighed. But she felt hopeful that she could help him to help himself. She couldn't heal the wounds. She knew that, but she could create the therapeutic environment in which his own psychological healing process might help him to recover. For these configurations within his self structure to have developed to the point of apparent independent existence as voices in his head, he must have been really affected, had he been young enough to maybe have dissociated in the experience? She wondered about this. They seemed sufficiently independent, and he may have been young enough to have developed this capacity to survive psychologically or cope with the trauma . . .

Her heart went out to him as a little boy, on his own, trying to cope with issues that the adults of the world can't resolve – what does a child do? Internalise, dissociate, create parts of yourself to hold the traumatised feelings or places to escape to. Psychological growth is disturbed, disrupted and distorted. And then the psychological problems begin. At least the foundations are established for symptoms to emerge that may seem so difficult to understand, and which may get pathologised by a diagnosis. Charlotte thought how we need to treat people beyond their symptoms, beyond the patterns of thought, feeling and behaviour that are simply the effects of underlying causes.

Summary

In counselling session 7 Ali talks more openly about his past and begins a process of recognising that there are parts to him that make up who he is, and he begins to identify them. They are more associated with particular behaviours than anything else. He plans to go away and map them out. However, this does not happen. Ali has had a difficult week, clashing with his father. In session 8 an exploration of this leads to an apparent 'psychotic' episode when Ali hear's voices in his head urging him to leave the session and smash something. He does not act on it and further exploration leads Ali to a deeper appreciation of that part of himself that he then calls 'jailbreak'; the part that wants to break free and get away. He draws this diagrammatically and then adds another part, 'hide away'. He finds himself getting calmer. Charlotte reflects after the session about the processes that can leave people with the kind of fragmented sense of self that Ali is experiencing.

Points for discussion

- Assess the quality of Charlotte's empathic responses in these two sessions.
- How do you react to the developing perception by Ali of the different 'parts' of himself?
- How would you feel if a client began hearing voices in the middle of a counselling session?
- What do you understand by the label/diagnosis 'psychotic'? If you received a referral from someone and the referral mentioned 'psychotic tendencies', how would you react?
- Some professionals suggest you need specific training to work with 'psychotic' clients. Is it a matter of training, or personal development? Discuss.
- If you were working as an independent practitioner with Ali, at what point would you feel it would be necessary to discuss his case with the other healthcare professionals involved in his treatment?

- The idea of treating causes rather than simply focusing on symptoms is raised in Charlotte's thinking at the end of session 8. Is this practical? How might services need to be shaped to respond to both underlying causes and symptomatic effects?
- Write your own notes for these sessions.

CHAPTER 8

Supervision session: Thursday 25th June – working at the edge of awareness

Charlotte had discussed her work with Ali on previous occasions with her supervisor, Matt. He had experience of working in a substance misuse setting with clients who had been diagnosed with mental health problems. He understood the nature and working of statutory services. Indeed, it was his experience of working in these areas that had been a major factor in Charlotte approaching him to be her supervisor. He not only supervised her work at the drug and alcohol service, but also her counselling work elsewhere.

Charlotte had been discussing one of her other clients and the theme of working with clients whose structure of self seems to be very fragmented emerged. Charlotte commented on the challenges of this, of being able to keep her own focus.

'Of course, once we begin to accept the notion that within the structure of self there are areas of specific identity, groupings of thoughts, feelings and behaviours along the lines of configurations within the self, then we must also accept the notion that we, as counsellors, as well as our clients, are subject to this reality. We often speak of clients in this context, but the counsellor or therapist will have their configurations – although personal development work should have enabled them to identify these and have perhaps more fully integrated them if there are signs of them being unduly separated from each other.'

Charlotte nodded as she listened to Matt. She was in agreement with him. 'The problem as I see it for the counsellor is when a "part" of himself or herself gets, in effect, hooked by a "part" of the client, and the counsellor is unaware that this is happening because they haven't got the necessary self-awareness to identify this process.'

Matt smiled. Yes, he knew that one as well. 'I agree. That is why I think training courses should have a large self-development focus, and I don't mean simply one-to-one therapy. In fact, I think very often the main focus should be within the training programme, through encounter, allowing these processes to be identified and used as material for the training and development process. Things get taken to a therapist that emerge from the training process and can end up becoming invisible to the trainers and the trainees' colleagues. From my experience, training as a person-centred counsellor meant a lot of personal development, and processing of experience within the training context, and that seemed to be the main focus. In fact, I was lucky, I had what I would call a person-centred training to become a person-centred counsellor, and that isn't always what happens. For me it again comes back to this notion of focusing more on how we are with out clients than what we do with them.'

The supervisor makes an interesting point. What balance should there be between theory, practice and personal development on counselling and psychotherapy training courses? With an approach that is so centred on the therapeutic relationship and the counsellor's ability to offer consistent empathy, unconditional positive regard and congruence, it is arguably even more important to have a strong focus on personal development within the training programme.

'A person-centred training puts the person of the individual therapist-to-be at the heart of the training process. This is consistent with a client-centred approach to therapy, which puts the client at the centre of the process, and with Rogers' belief that the person of the therapist is significant in the therapeutic process' (Embleton Tudor *et al.*, 2004, p. 64). Later, the authors highlight how 'training courses from different traditions pay different levels of attention to student's personal development' (Embleton Tudor *et al.*, 2004, p. 64). Indeed, with increasingly academic syllabuses the danger is that therapy training is moving more and more into knowledge and doing, and is at risk of sliding inexorably further and further away from being, from facilitating a would-be counsellor into becoming the congruent person who seeks to offer unconditional positive regard and convey empathic understanding to the client, whose values are naturally and congruently expressed through their practice and their presence within the therapeutic relationship. As the same authors suggest 'a person-centred training ... sees that the personal development of the student *is* the training, and for this reason gives it the highest priority' (Embleton Tudor *et al.*, 2004, p. 64).

'It comes back to congruence, to the counsellor knowing themselves well enough to be fully present with their client. To know the processes within themselves and their style of working. If I'm sitting in a session, listening to a client going through an intense experience, I need to be able to feel that I am clear on why I may be reacting in a particular way – whether it is my "stuff", as it were, my own conditioned reactions to something being discussed or a particular behaviour being exhibited before me, or whether I am in some way picking up on something specific to the client's process. As if someone says something and I may feel an urge to say something in response that is not an empathic response, but is something that becomes alive within me. Is it coming from a "part" of me that is conditioned into a certain perspective and reaction to what is occurring, or is it something other that may have specific meaning to the client and which, in a sense, the client is drawing out of me?'

'Can you say a little more, or give an example?'

'Yes, well, sort of. This may not be a good example, but perhaps it is. Ali, the client who has been using cannabis and has had an episode in hospital following what seemed to be some kind of psychotic disturbance. You know who I mean?'

Matt nodded. Yes, he remembered him from previous supervision sessions. He had already triggered interesting discussions between them around the whole issue of defining effective treatment responses for people so diagnosed. 'Mhmm.' He didn't say anymore, wanting to leave Charlotte to pursue her own train of thought.

'Well, in the last session, he. . . . No, let me put it in context. We had begun looking at his nature in terms of "parts" in a previous session. And he had gone away to identify the parts of himself. But there had been a problem at home that had upset him – his father can get on to him – and he had smashed a vase and, well, it had really got to him. But it also contributed to him later, in the session, relating to parts of himself. But anyway, what happened was he had a, well, I guess some would call it a "psychotic experience" in the last session.'

Matt frowned, unsure what Charlotte meant, and immediately experienced a sense of concern both for Charlotte and for Ali 'Were you OK with what happened, and Ali?'

'Yes, yes, but what was interesting was that, well, it turned out he was sitting there with voices in his head telling him to leave, to shut up, and to go and smash something. Now, he was sitting there, and he talked a bit to himself, and I responded something like commenting on how scary it must be for him to be experiencing what was happening for him. Now, he hadn't mentioned being scared. Was my response a genuine sensing of something present for him that I was picking up on, or was it part of me feeling scared by what I sensed was happening? At the time, well, it seemed to be scary for him, and I felt that what I was saying was a kind of expression of empathy, hoping to help him tell me what was happening, helping him to sense my own presence, I guess.'

'Mhmm, so you wanted to reach out and let him know you were there in a supportive kind of way?'

'But I didn't say that, I mean, I'd already said something about him taking his time, I only wanted to understand. But I could have said, "I'm here for you when you feel able to talk about it", but I introduced the scariness.'

'Did he look scared?'

'No, anxious, intense.' Charlotte tried to think back to the moment that it had happened. 'Like he was fighting with himself, or maybe that's a projection because I know what he talked about afterwards. No, he looked as though he was struggling with something.'

'So, Ali looks as though he is struggling with something, and you seek to reach out to him with an emphasis on it being scary, yes?'

Charlotte took a deep breath and sighed. 'Yes, I did. I didn't respond to the struggle, I noticed it but it got lost. And I brought in the scariness. And it was then that he began to knock his clenched fists together,' she demonstrated the movement, 'faster and faster. We didn't really explore that, in fact I applied pre-therapy responses as it really felt as though he had moved out of psychological contact. When he came back in contact with me he talked about there being this voice in his head. He seemed to be trying to focus himself. But where did the idea of scariness come from?'

'What do you think, given what we were saying earlier?'

'Maybe part of me feels scared witnessing the kind of struggle that was happening for Ali. Maybe something about him made some part of me feel scared, but my reality in that moment was not one of feeling scared myself.'

'OK, so the question is then whether within you there is a part of you that carries scariness in association with this kind of experience, but you are not in conscious touch with that part, but it can communicate?'

However much training, therapy and personal development work is undertaken, there remains the possibility that there will be areas within the counsellor that have not been fully explored. The counsellor, however experienced, has to remain open to the possibility that they will uncover aspects of themselves which were previously unknown. It is for this reason that becoming a person-centred counsellor is to enter on a journey of life-long learning.

Charlotte frowned as she thought about this, and its meaning. She could feel herself struggling with the idea that there were parts of herself that she was not aware of. She must be aware of them. She was an experienced therapist, but did she really know herself? Were there still blind spots? She didn't like the idea. She didn't like the idea of not having . . . the word 'control' came to mind. Not having control, not knowing what was going on inside herself. That felt scary. The notion of scariness wasn't a thought, it was a feeling that was suddenly very present for her.

Matt noted a change in Charlotte's expression. It suddenly looked very serious. He responded to what he saw. 'The way you look appears to me very serious.'

Charlotte felt slightly spaced out in herself. Something was happening inside her. She knew she had to explore it. 'I'm in a place where the thought of not knowing what is within my structure of self, and of therefore not feeling in control of who I am, well, that feels scary.' She looked across at Matt. 'Scary.'

Matt nodded. 'Mhmm. Scary to not feel in control.'

'For me, for me it's scary. May not be for someone else, though it probably should be, but for me it is scary. I have to own that and be aware that I actually feel that quite intensely. And yet it isn't something I feel generally. I . . .' She thought back to that last session with Ali. 'Is it around his mental state, the fact that he has been diagnosed as being psychotic? Is that heightening my sense of no control and triggering my own anxiety? Is it anxiety?' She thought about it, allowing the feeling to become more present. It was in her solar plexus region, a deep sense of unease. She nodded. 'I am uneasy about this.' Charlotte paused again. 'It feels like a kind of edge.'

'Edge?'

Charlotte nodded again but remained deep in thought. What did she mean by 'edge'? 'Like being close to something other, something unknown, something, yes, something. . .' She couldn't find a word that seemed to fit. Alien – no, that didn't sound right. Edge, edge of what?

Matt noted the frown still on Charlotte's face. He knew she was trying to work it through for herself. He respected her own internal processing and waited for when she was ready to communicate whatever it was she was experiencing.

'Edge. What do we mean by an edge? It's a boundary, a point or a line at which something ends and something else begins, perhaps? Or maybe it's like the edge on a horizon, it isn't that something ends and something else begins, it's the same continuum but it's out of sight. Out of sight . . . So.' Charlotte paused, trying to draw her thoughts together. 'So, something about being aware of an edge brings a sense of scariness to me.' She thought again as a fresh train of thought emerged for her. Edges and boundaries. She felt she was a well-boundaried therapist. She kept her boundaries, it was a professional requirement. She took a deep breath. 'Sorry, I'm in here processing. It's just triggered another line of thought for me.'

'Go on.'

'Well, edges are boundaries, and I feel I do keep boundaries, that it's one of my strengths.'

'Mhmm, I would agree with that, Charlotte.'

'And I see it as a professional requirement, something that I do and maintain as part of my professionalism.'

'Sure, your clear boundaries are you being professional.'

'Yes, but what if they aren't?'

It was Matt's turn to frown. 'Sorry, you mean, what if your boundaries are unprofessional?' He was unclear.

'No, the boundaries are professional but the motivation for having them isn't.'

'You mean your reasons for having boundaries are for reasons other than professionalism?'

Charlotte nodded. 'Supposing my boundaries are not being driven by professional need but by personal need. I need clear boundaries. I need to know where the edge is so I can keep away from it because to get too close, or to even think too much about what's over the edge, as it were, is too scary.'

Matt breathed deeply and sat back slightly. 'Right, I've got you. So you wonder whether your clear "boundariedness" is being motivated by your own personal feelings about being too close to an edge?'

'And the risk of not being in control that is associated with going over that edge, or beyond it. The idea of a horizon was one of the things that came to mind just now, of how a horizon appears to be an edge and yet it isn't really. But the thought that it is makes it something that can provoke anxiety if you thought you might have to go close to that edge.'

'Probably stopped ancient mariners exploring too far in case they fell off the world.'

'Right. So does my concept of an edge – and this feels scary, but a different kind of scary – does my concept of an edge in terms of human experience stop me from exploring?'

'Your edge, or the client's edge?'

Charlotte's immediate reaction was her own edge, but she hesitated. No, it wasn't just the client's edge, it was hers as well. 'Both, either. Any edge. Getting close to an edge in my own understanding or knowledge, or a client being on an edge that seemed to be getting close to my experiential horizon maybe? I haven't thought this through. But there is something about edges being scary, and coming back to what I was saying, does my being good with boundaries emerge out of my anxiety around edges more than my professionalism?' Another deep breath. She looked searchingly towards Matt. 'It's a big one, isn't it?'

Matt nodded, and was aware that he hadn't really had this discussion before, either about himself or with supervisees. And yet it seemed suddenly to have such relevance as an issue.

'It feels big, and makes me think of me as well. So, there is something then, perhaps, about what happened with Ali in that session that took you to a sense of an edge, provoked somewhere, somehow, a sense of scariness which, at the time, you were not conscious of, but which contributed to you responding to him in such a way that you highlighted the idea that it must be scary for him even though he was actually looking serious and concentrated?'

Charlotte listened and reflected on what Matt was saying. It sounded like a really good summary. She wished she could be clear like that, sometimes. 'And in a way, well, the session moved on and we got into exploring what the voices said, and he was able to identify a part in himself which he called "jailbreak", which is about wanting to get away, break free.'

Matt nodded, aware that Charlotte had moved on whilst he felt that there was a need to stay further with the topic of edges and boundaries, scariness and anxiety. The incident in the session may not have been in any way damaging for the therapeutic process, but it had opened up an area requiring exploration for Charlotte.

'OK, so the session moved on. But I'm still with the notion of the edge provoking unexperienced but communicated scariness, if that was what was happening for you.'

Charlotte put her hand across her mouth, resting her elbow on her other hand as she thought about it. She held her breath as she reflected further. 'Maybe I'm not as comfortable working with a client presenting with the kind of experiences that Ali has as I thought I was. Deep down, maybe I am uneasy about working at...' She pondered a phrase that came to mind, '... working at the psychotic edge. And having said that, you know, I want to unsay it because I don't, fundamentally, believe in that diagnosis in the sense that it's a social construct, like the horizon. No, well, the horizon's not a social construct but the meaning we attribute to it is.'

'Something about the meaning of "psychotic edge"?'

'If human beings, well. . .' Charlotte couldn't quite think of how to say what she was thinking. Her sense was that people extended beyond their normal selves. She didn't like the word normal, another social construct. 'Acceptable and unacceptable thinking, there's a boundary. It's OK to have a feeling to act in a particular way, a kind of hunch, but when it's a voice in your head telling you to do it then it becomes unacceptable. But it's a continuum, that's how I see it. So, I may have a kind of hunch or an urge to, say, go to the beach. That's fine. Quite normal and acceptable. But it could be that there is something else more urgent to attend to, but I still act on the inner urge. Well, still acceptable, but maybe it could be questioned. Perhaps I am meeting a stronger need to get away from something, either way I am now acting in a manner that is perhaps out of phase with what needs to be done. But generally that's still OK. But if I have a voice telling me to go to the beach, or commanding me to go, when there is something else to attend to, what then? It begins to become more unacceptable.'

'To whom?'

'I guess others who may be thinking, "Why did she do that when she needed to do this?".'

'OK.'

'And then the next extreme is the voice telling someone to do something that is harmful to themselves or others. Then it becomes a mental health problem, at least, that's how it seems to be. It's OK to have voices, but not if they tell you to act bizarrely or in an antisocial way.'

'So it is the content of the voice and the nature of the behaviour that defines whether the person is on a psychotic edge?'

'But it could be normal to them. I guess the extreme situations where people are at risk to themselves or others, yes, that needs addressing for reasons of safety and risk. But if there is no risk or safety issue, but say someone hears a voice telling them, I don't know, to spend their life feeding pigeons because that is what God wants them to do, and they hear God's voice very clearly. It's a daft example, but no one is being harmed. Is that psychotic? Or is that someone who likes birds, wants to feel good about caring for birds, and they have created a way of giving themselves permission to do this?'

'Mhmm, not sure where you are going, but OK.'

'Neither am I, but it is something about, for me, the idea of a psychotic edge. Part of me feels that it is a construct, it's inconsistent, and yet there are severely disturbed people who clearly live beyond my horizon, who experience things which trigger behaviours that are outside my knowledge and understanding. People who, if you like, are over my edge.'

Matt smiled. 'And that's the crucial factor. Who's edge? Who defines the edge? For you, working with a client, it is your edge that matters in terms of your ability to be a companion with that client, yes? That's what we have to deal with. Yes, the broader debate remains. But in therapy, as a counsellor, can you define your edge and can you work with people who are close to or over that edge?'

'And that's about professional and personal competence?'

'Yes.'

Charlotte suddenly felt clearer. 'This is really helping. Getting this out, exploring, just going through this process. I've not talked like this before, it is helpful. I have to define my edge. And in that session Ali was on that edge and maybe over it, and so I have to extend my horizon.'

'He's helping you do that, in a way. The question is when he invites you into his world, beyond your horizon, can you take that journey with him and still be able to get back into the world this side of it?'

Charlotte nodded, but somehow the idea didn't feel as scary as it had done before. Now she had a metaphor, no, it was more than a metaphor, a framework within which to operate. She could maintain professional boundaries for professional reasons, but her own psychological and emotional boundaries needed to be more open, and she needed to be at ease with that.

'I really appreciate this. This discussion and exploration, well, it has itself extended my horizon, it really has. And it all happened through this process. My calmness in the session may have been sort of false, but my anxiety emerged through my reference to it being scary for Ali. Perhaps I can now experience more of a genuine calmness and also a clearer connection with my own sense of the scariness – my scariness – of sailing close to the edge. I'm back to the ancient explorers wondering if they'd fall off the edge of the world.'

'And it was a reasonable view in the context of the knowledge and understanding of the time.'

'I wonder how our current ideas around mental health will be viewed in the future when we travel beyond our current horizon in our treatment and understanding of mental health problems, and, of course, substance use?'

The focus of the supervision moved on to another client. For both Charlotte and Matt it had been a valuable dialogue, extending themselves as they grappled with the notion of working with clients who exist close to an edge, and the impact that this can have on the counsellor.

Counselling session 9: Tuesday 30th June – paranoia in the session

The supervision session had had a profound effect on Charlotte. She did feel somehow more extended. It was hard to really describe what she was feeling, but she sensed very clearly a difference. She was not sure how it would impact on her work with Ali, or any of her other clients. Those that she had seen since the supervision session were not going through the kind of intense experiences that Ali was having. She had spent a lot of time after that supervision session thinking. She often gave herself space after supervision, deliberately timing it so, if the weather was fine, she could go and sit outside somewhere to reflect, or if the weather was bad, sit somewhere quiet with tea and a cake.

Being able to make visible the idea of having an edge in a sense seemed to have helped diminish it, or maybe dissolve it, or even more likely, as with the horizon, as she moved towards it without fear of falling over the edge she was able to appreciate how it moves further away, allowing for extended awareness. And maybe that was what had happened. She had been able to move closer to the idea of her edge which enabled her horizon to extend. She hoped it would help her to be more fully present for Ali, more self-aware and more able to be a companion in his inner world.

She also wondered how her own – and the word that had come to mind was an interesting one – how her own perhaps 'edginess', even though she may not have been conscious of it, may have impacted on Ali and his ability to feel free to be how he needed to be in the sessions.

The intercom on the phone disturbed her thoughts. 'Your client's arrived.'

'Thanks.' Charlotte took a deep breath and brought her focus back. She was interested to see how she would be, but she was also mindful of not spending so much time watching herself so that it blocked her responsiveness to Ali.

Ali came in. He looked preoccupied. His expression wasn't relaxed, he looked drawn and his head movements seemed jerky. He stared at the door after they had sat down. Charlotte did not know what was happening for him and she was aware of her own edginess emerging. She recognised it, acknowledged it and took a deep breath. She thought to herself: I have to go into his world, I have to be prepared to approach my horizon. She thought of the image of the sea – she had pondered this after the supervision session. She would need to sail out to where Ali was, even if it risked heading towards the horizon, beyond which existed the unknown and the risk of falling over the edge. She knew, however, there was no edge, not really, but a continuum.

'Where are you Ali?' She sought to ascertain his position in order to reach out to him.

'She's listening, you know? They are all listening.'

'Listening to . . . ?'

'To my thoughts, to what I say, what we say. They never stop listening.' He continued to stare at the door.

'They're listening now?'

Ali did not nod, he just continued to stare. He closed his eyes. Ali believed he was being heard, that his thoughts were being read, he knew it and, at the same time, some part of him also knew that it wasn't true, but that part was lost to his awareness. 'I don't trust them.' He turned to stare towards Charlotte. It unnerved her for a moment or two. Again, the thought returned for her – he's near your edge, your horizon, reach out to where he is.

'You don't trust them because they listen to you?'

Ali said nothing. He could hear them listening to him. He could feel them reading his thoughts. There was nowhere to hide. He wanted a joint. He needed a joint. He'd been OK when he left home, but he'd caught the bus over and there were people laughing and joking and he heard someone say his name. It wasn't that he knew any of them, but he became convinced they were talking about him. The journey lasted about 20 minutes and he heard his name on other occasions. It wound him up. They knew who he was, they had been waiting for him to get on the bus, they knew he was going to get on, they knew where he was going, they probably still knew what he was thinking.

Charlotte noted no change in Ali's expression following her response. Was he aware of her? Was there psychological contact?

Once again the counsellor is faced with the possibility that her client may have moved outside of psychological contact. She does not know if her presence, or anything she is saying, is being registered by her client.

'Ali, can you hear me?'

Ali continued to stare. He heard Charlotte's voice but it seemed distant, far from the thoughts in his head. He heard her speak again, this time it was a little clearer. Charlotte had raised her voice a little.

Ali blinked. 'Mhmm, yeah?'

'Hi Ali, it's OK, you seemed to go distant there for a while.'

He looked anxious, 'Yeah, they knew my name, they were listening to me.'

'Mhmm, can you tell me who they were?'

'Don't know them, they were on the bus.'

'Mhmm, on the bus, and they knew your name?'

'Yes, I heard them talk about me.'

'You heard them talk about you.'

'Yeah, they were talking about me, saying my name. They were saying lots of things about me.'

'Saying lots of things about you.' Charlotte sought to ensure her emphasis and intonation matched Ali's.

'Yeah, and reading my thoughts, seeing inside my head.'

'Reading your thoughts, seeing inside your head.'

'Yeah.'

Ali lapsed into silence. He felt extremely anxious, wished he'd gone home.

Charlotte kept to very simple responses, focusing on what Ali was saying. It wasn't that she did not have psychological contact now, she did not need to use pre-therapy responses. But she kept it simple nonetheless. 'Yeah. That's how it was.'

'They kept saying things.' Ali looked suddenly more anxious.

'What did they say about you?'

'They said ... I don't know, but they were talking about me and laughing and looking at me.'

'Mhmm, so they used your name, yes, and did they say your whole name?'

'They said "Ali". I heard them talking about me.'

'Mhmm. Ok, they talked about Ali, yes?'

'Yes, they were waiting for me.'

'Waiting for you, on the bus?'

Ali nodded. It was his first body movement for a while.

'So they waited for you and you heard someone say "Ali"?'

'Yes.'

'And you thought they were talking about you?'

'They were, I heard them, they were laughing and looking at me.'

'So you were sitting close to them when you heard them?'

'I was a few seats in front of them. They were laughing at me.'

'Laughing at you. That must have been very uncomfortable.'

'Hated it, always hate being laughed at.'

'Always hate being laughed at. Something you've experienced before?'

'At school, they laugh at me. They laugh and make fun of me. They call me names, hate it, hate them, hate them all.'

Charlotte noted the shift of focus. Ali was talking about school now and had switched to a present tense.

It is likely that Ali has switched into a part of himself that developed out of his childhood experience. Being laughed at has taken him to the part of himself that he developed and went to in the past when it happened. Charlotte keeps her focus on what he is saying, careful not to introduce anything new. Part of Ali is speaking, and it has probably not had much opportunity to speak. She needs to ensure she offers that part the warm acceptance and empathy she would offer Ali as a whole, or any other part that presented itself.

'They laugh and make fun of you at school, call you names, and you hate it, all of it.' Charlotte kept the focus and kept to the present tense. She wasn't sure what was happening for Ali but she thought that maybe he was connecting with some deeply affected part of himself that had its origin in the school experience but which had been triggered by the experience on the bus.

'All the time. I hate it. Hate it.'

'You hate being laughed at and called names. Hate it.'

Ali nodded. He was listening to himself speaking and he felt somewhat detached from himself, as though he was watching himself or hearing himself speak. He took a deep breath. He felt a bit light-headed. He blinked and moved his neck.

'Where are you now, Ali?'

'Here, sitting on this chair.'

'OK, so you hate being laughed at at school, and you hated it on the bus earlier?'

'Yes. They talk about me, everyone talks about me.'

'I really hear you saying that, Ali, it really feels like everyone is talking about you.'

'No one believes me, but you do, don't you?'

'I believe that you experience people talking about you, Ali. It happened at school, for real. And you hated it. And now when it happens, or you think it happens, like on the bus, it really affects you.'

This is an unhelpful response – it does not convey genuine acceptance of what Ali is experiencing and the way that he is interpreting it. It is a supervision issue for Charlotte, if she notes it as having happened, to check out her need to respond in the way that she has, and to step out of Ali's frame of reference and therefore cloud her empathy.

'You don't think they were listening to me?'
'I wonder if maybe one of them was called Ali, and you may have thought they were talking about you.'

The counsellor is trying to challenge Ali's experience. Charlotte, having stepped away from a client-centred focus, is now trying to rationalise an experience that essentially is irrational to her frame of reference although, of course, within Ali's frame of reference it makes perfect sense and is therefore quite rational. Her challenge naturally arouses his anxiety and he defends himself. He has to. The thought that his experience is false, when he is expressing himself through the part of him that believes it to be true, is too difficult to bear. It could leave him feeling unable to express that part of his experience to Charlotte and the therapeutic opportunity for him to feel heard and understood, and to explore in his own way and pace will be lost.

At this time, it may be that Ali might be described as psychotic, but whether or not this label applies, he is in psychological contact with Charlotte. They are communicating in a meaningful way, though it's simply that what Ali is experiencing and believing within his frame of reference is outside of what is acceptable within Charlotte's frame of reference. She has to work at staying with him, however much she might find what he is describing hard to believe. Ali is describing his world, his experience. The person-centred counsellor empathises and warmly accepts. Whilst some might suggest this will simply collude and reinforce, the person-centred viewpoint will be that the part that needs to believe that it is talked about, listened to, spied upon, is perhaps fragile, vulnerable and deeply traumatised. Gentle, warm acceptance can help that part to feel valued and accepted, and a process of re-integration may begin to take place; the person's structure of self having less need to 'split' off the hard-to-accept feelings.

Why is this important? Because the part that is speaking is traumatised, it didn't get heard in the past or perhaps wasn't able to speak. The boy who was taunted, picked on, who knew that the other kids did talk about him, has grown and developed and has now extended this into his young adult experiences. It needs to be heard and the only way that this can happen is for the counsellor to continue to empathise with what it needs to say.

Ali shook his head. He suddenly seemed very agitated again.

'OK, that's really hard to accept right now, yes?'

'They were spying on me, like our neighbours, they do that, they listen through the wall, I hide in my room, I hide in the smoke, but they can still hear me.'

'They listen to you as well.'

'No one believes me. Mum doesn't believe me. She tells me that it's in my head, but it isn't. I know. I hear them.'

'You hear them and they are listening to you.'

Charlotte was aware that she was feeling totally confused and a little spaced out. She was wondering whether Ali would come out of his current state of mind. His world wasn't making sense but it was his world. She decided to stay with it, stay with him, maintain her empathy and unconditional positive regard wherever it took her, took them.

'I'm always being listened to, being spied on. They want to know what's in my head.'

'Mhmm, always listened to and spied on, always wanting to know what's in your head.'

'I try to stop them. The spliffs help but I can't have them any more. I try to distract myself like Desmond tells me, but that doesn't always work. I want them to stop.'

'Sounds like you really try, you really want them to stop.' It sounded to Charlotte that the part of Ali that knew he needed to fight against these kind of thoughts was emerging. Perhaps the paranoia was beginning to ease.

Ali is now expressing himself through another part of himself. It is the part that fights against the paranoia taking over, that knows it is not true, that seeks to apply the ideas and techniques that Desmond has suggested.

Ali closed his eyes and tried to focus. The intensity was easing. He opened his eyes and looked at Charlotte. 'I don't want to feel watched and spied on, I don't. I don't like people looking at me. I want to hide. Makes me go crazy. Makes me want to hide.'

Charlotte nodded. 'Yes. I can only imagine how awful it must be for you, Ali. Wanting to get away from it all, wanting to hide away, feeling crazy with it.' She kept her voice quiet and calm.

'I want to be normal, I want to not think these things. I try not to. I talk to Desmond. I try to keep in control, but things happen and it all gets out of control again.'

Ali suddenly burst into tears, deep, racking sobs. It took Charlotte totally by surprise. She hadn't somehow expected Ali to cry in a session, but here he was, crying in front of her, tears streaming down his cheeks. Something had burst out of him, something was being released. She didn't disturb him, but kept her focus. 'Let it go, let it out.' She again spoke gently, not wanting to disturb or distract Ali from the emotional release that was occurring for him.

'I know that it's in my head,' Ali swallowed and took a tissue. 'I know that but I can't stop myself sometimes. It gets out of control and I think everyone's talking about me. I know they're not, but at the time, I know that they are.'

'Yes, you know that they're not but there are times when you think that they are.'

'The puff used to control it. At least, that's how it felt. But now it's really difficult sometimes and I lose it. I must have seemed crazy earlier.'

Charlotte smiled. 'Let's say you seemed to be in another place, but no, not crazy.'

'You know, the parts we talked about, there's a crazy me, it's me when I get paranoid. I go to some crazy place and it's so real. I can just suddenly be there. I wasn't thinking like that on my way over, but the bus trip was what got to me. I don't know why. It was a bit busy but not too bad. Just hearing my name, you know?'

'Yes, hearing your name and seeing them looking your way and laughing.'

'And it was like when I was at school. But then they used to call me names as well, and laugh and stare, and I was so miserable, really, really miserable. My life was a nightmare.'

'Mhmm, and so whilst you sometimes get it in your head that people are talking about you when they're not, the reality is in childhood that they were.'

Ali was nodding. 'Yeah. Yeah. I know it happens, and then I lose it and think it's still happening, and...' He shook his head, feeling utter despair at himself. 'It's so difficult because when it's happening it all feels OK, well, not OK because it makes me so edgy, but it is OK as well because I know they're listening.' He shook his head and closed his eyes. 'And I know they're not, but not when it's happening.'

'So it's OK and not OK – OK because they're listening and not OK because you feel edgy. You know it isn't happening but at the time it is, it feels so real.'

Ali nodded. He took a deep breath and sighed.

Charlotte nodded slowly, tight-lipped, really unsure what to say. Somehow it felt like there wasn't anything to say. Ali had said how it was and she had heard him and had confirmed that what she was hearing was how he wanted to describe his experience.

Ali was still nodding. He sighed again. 'But I don't want to be like that, not any more. I want to be normal, but I get anxious when I go out sometimes. I get anxious in big places, and when it's busy.'

'The anxiety stops you going out?'

'Stops me doing things. Makes it difficult sometimes to go out. I just feel so on edge. Smoking a joint or two always calmed me down. It's really hard now. I do still have one now and then, but it's so hard to cope without it.'

'So, it's hard without the joints not to feel anxious.' Charlotte paused. 'Have you talked to Desmond about this because he might be able to work on this with you?' She was thinking of how his cognitive-behavioural approach might help Ali to work at slowly adjusting to the kind of situations that at the moment made him feel anxious.

Why has Charlotte suddenly introduced Desmond and the work he is doing? She has taken Ali right out of his frame of reference to something in hers. She had no need to add anything to her initial empathic response. And she hasn't recognised what she has done. In a sense she is out of touch with herself as a person-centred counsellor, a part of her that perhaps wants someone to fix it for Ali. If she was aware of what she had done she could take it to supervision, but she isn't. It's a blind spot. This situation highlights the value of sometimes recording sessions (with the client's consent) to listen to later, or to take to supervision. Effectively, Charlotte has rescued Ali from his anxiety and the focus is now on calming him down.

'A bit. Something to calm me down would help.'
'You can be calmed down, I remember how you were after that relaxation, the first time in particular.'

Is Charlotte manipulating the session – albeit unwittingly – in order to offer a relaxation? If so, and given what has happened, the question might be asked of who it is actually for. Perhaps Charlotte at some level is feeling overwhelmed by the session, by what has been happening, and she is looking for a break. The problem is that she is unaware, she cannot therefore be considered to be being congruent.

Ali could still remember that. 'I'd like to do that again. It really did help. Maybe I need to do that more often. I need to be able to do it myself.'
'Have you any relaxing music?'
'Not really. You think I should get something?'
'Do you think it would help?'
'Don't know. I wish I could do that relaxation more often, it really helped.'
'Maybe we could do it to end the session today.'
'Yes, I'd really like that. I think I need it.'
'OK.' Charlotte checked the time. 'Well, we could use the last ten minutes. What about the time before then?'
'I want to go back to the drawing from last week. I want to add a crazy or paranoid part of me to it.'
'OK.' Charlotte had it on the table and passed it over to Ali. He added it in, putting it in a bubble that extended outside of his head. 'This is because when I go crazy I kind of think things are happening outside my head. It's not just me, it's what I think others are doing. I kind of go out of my head.'
'So, there's "jailbreak", "hide away" and now "crazy, paranoid", which goes outside of your head, yes?'

'I also get low as well, and sad. There's a sad and lonely me as well.' Another
   bubble. 'Not much more room in my head.'
'That also how it feels?'
Ali nodded. 'Yeah, too much. . .' He paused. 'There.'
'That's you?'
'So far. Probably more, but that's me. I'm sometimes one or other of these.'
'Always at least one of them?'
Ali looked at them and thought about it. 'When I smoke puff well I kind of feel I'm
   in "hide away". But I guess sometimes I'm none of them. But I do get anxious,
   you know, and panicky. Yeah, there's a kind of panicky me in there as well.
   I need to add that.' He wrote in 'panic' and drew another bubble around it in
   his head.
'So, you move around between them?'
'Yeah, and I don't like any of them except "Jailbreak". That's where I want to be.
   I want to break out.' The song was back in his head again. 'Yeah, I want to
   break out.'
'Break out.'
Ali went silent. He was still looking at what he had drawn. He felt sure there must
   be other bubbles in his head but it was complicated enough with what he'd
   already written. It made sense to him. 'So, what do I do about all of this?'
'What do you want to do?'

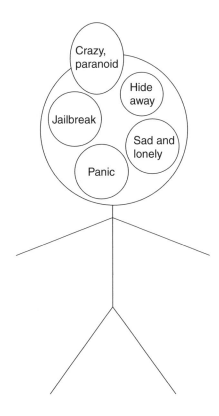

'Seems a bit less scary to see it written down. I mean, when it's happening it's like I don't know what's happening. It feels so out of control.'

'Out of control, yes, it just takes over.'

'But it's me, isn't it, I mean, these are parts of me, it's parts of me taking over?'

'Mhmm, how does that seem?'

'Makes sense but it doesn't always feel like that. It can feel like someone's telling me what to do, it really can.'

'Mhmm, so which ones feel like that?'

' "Jailbreak", like last time, voice telling me to get out of here. That feels sometimes in my head, but sometimes not.'

'Sometimes in your head, sometimes somewhere else?'

'It changes. Sometimes it can feel real close, but it can also be beside me or behind me. So I guess that bubble should be a bit outside of my head as well.' He changed the drawing.

'So, the voice that tells you to get out, get away, can seem as though it is in your head sometimes, but it can also feel like it is coming from outside of your head as well.'

'Same with feeling I want to hide away. Usually that feels in my head, but sometimes it seems outside. But not as often. That one's usually inside, telling me to hide away, usually telling me to smoke a joint.'

'So smoking a joint is linked to the "hide away" part.'

'Yeah, that's how it is.'

Having written and now amended the drawing, Ali is now refining it, and using it to convey to Charlotte his experience. And she is listening and accepting what he is saying about his experience. Ali is acknowledging them as parts of himself, although he also conveys his experience that at times they do not feel like parts of himself. What is emerging is quite a sophisticated dialogue, and not all clients will engage so fully in this process. This is an illustration of how an apparently psychotic experience can be made sense of, can be understood in the context of a client's inner experience. But there needs to be a capacity to self-reflect to achieve this. For some clients, much more time will be spent seeking to establish and hold some degree of psychological contact, particularly for the client who is more fully engaged with his inner, psychotic processes, who is moving through the different areas of his traumatically affected self-structure. And there will be some people whose structure of self is such that whilst there may be contact with the outer world, their processing of their experience requires the counsellor to stay with pre-therapy responses over a lengthy period of time in order to offer the opportunity of establishing some degree of relational contact and the possibility of the start of a healing process.

'OK, look, time for the relaxation if you want to do that again.'

'Yeah, I do.' Ali put the pencil down and pushed the paper away.

'Same as the first time?'

Ali nodded.

'OK. So, sit in a way that is comfortable and relax.' She went through the relaxation routine again, and once more Ali found it incredibly helpful. He really felt slowed down in himself.

Ali left the session without that edgy anxiety that was so familiar to him. He was grateful for that. It lasted for a while. It was when he got off the bus – he nearly missed his stop – that he felt the anxiety returning. By the time he was back home he was on edge again. His mother was home and asked him how he had got on. He told her about the session. He had spoken to her before about the counselling, but this time he said a lot more. She was still continuing with her own counselling and had been so glad that Ali had taken it up. They talked for quite a while and it helped Ali to feel a bit more settled once more. It seemed to somehow reinforce something that he was being listened to, that what he was saying was being accepted. Charlotte, Desmond, and now his mother, all seemed to accept what he was saying, and that somehow felt good, felt like a relief in some way.

Meanwhile, Charlotte was looking at the diagram Ali had drawn. She wondered, as she had before, how many other bubbles there might be. But there was no point in speculating. It was for Ali to discover what made up his structure of self. They had made a start. He had a kind of map and he seemed to be embracing this idea of different 'parts' within himself. She hoped it would make sense for him. She also knew that it wasn't only about thinking and theorising. She had seen some of these 'parts' emerge in the session and she knew that much of the important therapy would be connected with how she responded to these 'parts' in the sessions now and in the future, and maybe more 'parts' would emerge. Could Ali begin to create a stronger, conscious bridge between them, and perhaps modify some of them as he re-evaluated his life and the experiences that had shaped his structure of self? She felt good that she had stayed with Ali during his paranoia at the start of the session. She wondered how much the supervision had helped her in this. In truth, she did not know, but felt that it must have helped. She had stayed more centred, calmer, more accepting of the fact that she did not know what was happening in Ali's reality. She realised how challenging it is to trust a client's process when their process seems utterly outside of your own experience, or what may be decided by society to be 'normal'.

Summary

In supervision, Charlotte explores her thinking and feeling in relation to a sense of scariness that she introduced in a previous session. This leads into a discussion around the process of working with someone who is on an edge in themselves that may be outside of the experience and awareness of the counsellor.

In session 9, Ali arrives in a somewhat paranoid state, convinced people on the bus were talking about him. This slowly settles, and he returns to the diagram containing the different 'parts' of himself that he has identified. He adds 'crazy paranoid', 'sad and lonely' and 'panic'.

Points for discussion

- What is your reaction to the exploration that developed in the supervision session?
- Where is your 'edge' when it comes to working with people with mental and behavioural problems, and why is it positioned in that place? How might you extend it?
- How would you have responded to Ali coming into the session in a paranoid state?
- Can you identify any of the parts of Ali as having meaning within your own structure of self? If so, what of your thoughts, feelings and behaviours associated with them?
- Are there other parts of Ali that you think have emerged but were not included in the diagram?
- How effective was Charlotte in applying the core conditions in her responses to Ali?
- What do you think was happening when Charlotte took Ali's focus away from his anxiety and started talking about what Desmond could offer?
- Write your own notes for this session.

CHAPTER 9

Counselling session 10: Tuesday 7th July – Ali draws a 'map' of his structure of self

Charlotte was sitting in the counselling room waiting for Ali to arrive and wondering how he would be. She was glad that he had taken to the relaxation visualisation at the end of the session, it had seemed to help him. He was clearly living on an edge within himself and it seemed that it did not take much for him to feel perhaps in some sense overwhelmed. She wondered whether his having spent a lot of time in his room had affected him. Whether he was now very sensitive to noise and movement, stimulating or over-stimulating environments where there was a lot going on. She had seen this with clients in the past, particularly those who had used a lot of suppressive or sedating substances. They could feel so overwhelmed. How many people had she seen who could not bear large supermarkets, how they seemed so easily at the mercy of panic attacks.

She felt good that Ali was working with Desmond. He approached things in a different, yet complementary way. Like her, whilst he believed that some mental health problems were organic and needed a chemical intervention to help rebalance the processes in the brain, he also felt strongly that many problems stemmed from experiences in life. Desmond would work much more directly on the cognitive aspects, helping his clients to think differently about specific issues and events and to learn new behavioural responses. Whilst her emphasis was very much on the relational experience in therapy, offering the core conditions to help the client in a sense redefine themselves and re-integrate aspects of their nature that had become separated out to some degree – she thought of the different 'parts' that Ali had so far identified.

Combining different therapeutic or treatment approaches in this way should be researched. There are assumptions about how a client should only be in therapy with one therapist at any time, but on what is this assumption based? Where is the evidence base that two professionally skilled counsellors cannot work individually with the same client? In this case it is a counsellor and a community psychiatric nurse working with one client, applying contrasting cognitive-behavioural therapy (CBT) and person-centred approaches. In life we do not have just one relationship, we move between them. So long as the two approaches are not both characterised by techniques of telling the client what to do, which would be confusing to say the least should differences arise, then there is perhaps opportunity for complementarity. Are there situations in which a client having more than one therapeutic relationship is helpful?

It seems to me that one of the strengths of person-centred therapy is that it can be applied in conjunction with other kinds of intervention, but not at the same time by the same person. It can provide a setting for the client to explore more deeply what is happening for them as a result of the other intervention, whether it is CBT, medication, motivational work, 12-step programmes (Alcoholics Anonymous). This is not to question the necessary and sufficient nature of the person-centred approach, but necessary and sufficient does not imply that something else in conjunction with person-centred therapy might not be helpful.

It was time for Ali to arrive and Charlotte made her way out to the reception area. She arrived just as he was coming through the door. 'Hello Ali, come on through.'

Ali followed her. He was feeling a lot better in himself this week. Things had settled down again at home and he was feeling easier in himself. He had appreciated the way Charlotte had been with him the previous week, and the relaxation had helped again. He was keeping away from the cannabis and felt that the diagram he'd drawn the previous week had helped. The image had stayed with him. It didn't feel so scary and out of control now that he had a clear image in his mind of himself. He'd talked about it with Desmond and that had been valuable as well. It had left him again with a sense that perhaps he could control things a little better now.

'So, how do you want to use the time today?'

'I've had a better week and I've been thinking about those different "parts" of me. It seems to me that my problem is that I am either one thing or the other. I sort of jump around, can't seem to be in control of it sometimes, you know?'

Charlotte nodded. 'Jumping between the parts with little or no control.'

'And I want that control. I mean, I suppose I want to be able to . . . ,' he thought about it for a moment, unsure quite what he wanted, but he knew he didn't want to keep feeling he had no control. He looked at Charlotte and shrugged.

'You want control but you want something else but it's hard to know what that is?'

'It's like I . . . ,' again he paused. It was something about feeling more whole, but he wasn't sure quite what he meant by that. He tightened his lips and frowned. Another thought came to him. 'I know I want to feel calmer, not so anxious and edgy.'

Charlotte nodded in response and acknowledged what he had said. 'Feeling calmer, not so anxious and edgy. More settled?'

'Something like that. It does my head in the way I have been.' Charlotte noted the use of the past tense which she sensed as indicating that at least for now Ali was feeling in a different place in himself.

'The way you've been, did your head in, but it sounds like you feel different now.'

'I do. This week has been better. The last session seemed to help. The relaxation was really good again. But the more I think of myself in "parts", yes, and last week I really was being my paranoid self, and you listened, you stayed with me, and somehow that was really important. And I don't know why, and I don't understand it, but it seems to have helped a lot.'

'Sounds like the paranoid you doesn't often get listened to.'

'People back off. Or at least, well, maybe it's me, me backing off from them. That's probably the truth. Me backing off because, well, when I'm in that state I don't trust anyone.'

'So the paranoid part of you doesn't trust anyone?'

Ali shook his head. 'Makes me feel very alone as well. Like it's only me.' He took a deep breath. 'But you kind of changed that last week by listening, trying to understand me.' He breathed deeply. 'So,' he nodded to himself, 'so...' He didn't know what to say. He felt suddenly quite emotional. His eyes watered and he blinked.

'Only you, but that you felt heard, understood...' Charlotte didn't empathise with the emotion in his eyes, but rather to the comment that had seemed to have triggered it.

'I don't think I'm used to being listened to, not really. Maybe that's why I don't tell people things unless I feel I can trust them.'

'Trust's so important for you to be able to tell people things.'

Ali nodded but stayed silent.

Charlotte respected his silence and waited for him to continue.

> Silence is a form of communication and the empathic response to communicated silence is to respect that silence and communicate it back. In other words, the counsellor stays silent but remains focused and attentive on the client and on their own internal process. It may sound strange, it may not, but in silence sometimes the deepest quality of communication can be achieved.

Ali was thinking back, aware of how few people he really trusted. A few friends from over the years, and his mum. Yes, she did sometimes seem to get on his nerves, getting all anxious and worried about him, yet he knew deep down she cared, that she wanted the best for him. She'd always been the one trying to ensure he got help when he needed it. The days when his mood had really swung and at times he'd been really depressed. Now, well, she seemed to be easier to talk to. She seemed more ..., he wasn't sure how to describe it, but, well, it was like she was more confident and also more open and approachable, more relaxed maybe. He wasn't sure. But there was a difference and it felt easier. She didn't fuss around him so much. Yeah, she was concerned sometimes, and he knew he still preferred to withdraw and hide away. But he had had some good conversations with her recently about things, and about himself. She'd really listened. He reckoned that her going to counselling for herself must have helped, not that he wanted his mum for a counsellor, but it was good to talk to her. He felt closer to her now. Yeah, he thought, I trust her as well, but in a different way, maybe more like a mother.

Charlotte continued sitting quietly, being aware of her own reactions to the silence. It seemed to her that Ali wasn't being simply passive, or stuck for something to say. He seemed more lost in thought. She wondered how he would be when he emerged from his process. She didn't know and what was the point in speculating anyway. He would be how he needed to be and she must be sensitive and responsive.

Ali was shaking his head slightly. 'Don't think about the pot so much now. I mean I still do, but not as much. Haven't had any for a while now. Still not sure if I'm better off for it. Did seem to help me feel better.'

Charlotte nodded. 'Better in that it took you away from feelings?'

Ali nodded. 'And thoughts, and the voices in my head. Still kind of talk to myself, you know, silently, but that's not the same, is it?'

'Does it feel the same?'

'No. I feel more in control at the moment. But, well, I know something could set me off again. Get paranoid about something and want to hide away. Those two parts of me seem really linked, you know?'

'The paranoid you and the part that wants to hide away?'

'Yeah, but it also makes me go crazy as well. Never really know which it'll be. But I just want to be normal, like I've said before, kind of let things settle down a bit.'

'Mhmm, normal and settled.'

'Like in those relaxations.' He shook his head, still not really believing that he could experience such a calm simply from counting numbers and imagining a colour. 'They're really good.'

'You have that calmness within you, just has to be found.'

'I think I maybe need to add that "part" to the diagram.' He took the paper which Charlotte had put out in case Ali had wanted to add to it. He drew another bubble and just wrote 'calm' in it.

'Calm.' Charlotte spoke the word calmly. It somehow seemed appropriate.

Ali took a deep breath. 'Yeah, I need that. I wish I could get to it a bit more easily though, wish I had the control to do that.'

'Ability to take yourself into that calm place?'

Ali nodded. He thought of the relaxation and dropped his shoulders. He hadn't realised how tense they had been. 'I thought I was relaxed.'

'You seem to carry a lot of tension there.'

'Mum keeps telling me to relax. I pace around a bit sometimes at home. Nothing really slows me down any more, I mean, not like the pot.'

'So you find it hard to relax?'

'Can't switch my head off sometimes. It's not like the voices. They seem to have faded. Well, they were there last week, whenever it was. No, oh I don't know, I lose track of time. When I was feeling paranoid on the bus coming here, yeah, then the voices were there, but not so much since. I seem to be more in control, more able to divert my attention. And sometimes when I feel as though they're going to start I've learned to say "no" and do something. Desmond's really helped me with that.'

'Sounds like he's helped you but you are now doing it for yourself.' Charlotte responded in this way because she wanted to acknowledge that Ali was doing this for himself and that he could take encouragement from that perhaps.

'Guess I am.'

Charlotte smiled. 'Mhmm, seems that way to me.'

'But I'm not relaxing, I get thoughts in my head. I just keep thinking about things.'

'Thoughts just go round and round in your head?'

'I can't seem to stop them when they start. I mean, they're not big thoughts, but they won't stop.'

'Can you say what they are like?' Charlotte knew she had moved away from empathic responding the moment that she spoke.

It might be argued that the counsellor is helping to draw the issue out of the client, and this can have value, but it would not be person-centred practice. It would be leading and directing. Whilst, from a person-centred perspective, it is unfortunate that the empathic connection has been momentarily broken, at least the counsellor recognises it. It means that she may choose to process this. Perhaps it could lead her, in supervision, to realise that she is finding her client overwhelming at times, that his inner world is too big, perhaps too confusing, for her to stay in touch with. A more person-centred response would probably have been along the lines of, 'So these thoughts you can't seem to stop. It's not they are big, but they just won't stop. They sound like they just keep going.' Not exactly the same words, but they would have acknowledged what was being conveyed. Empathising to the same order in which the client has spoken is also important. Sometimes a client is changing their focus as they speak, or developing an idea or a feeling. It is important to empathise with the process as well.

'I replay events, thinking about what people have said, or about what they might think. I'm still very aware of people around me. I don't think about them the same as I did, but I'm very aware of them, and I wonder what they think of me, how I must have looked to them, whether they could see my anxiety, whether I should say something to them and, if I did, what would I say?'

'Replaying it all in your head.'

'I know a joint would stop it.'

'Mhmm, you sound pretty sure of that.'

'I am, I miss all that. But I've got to get used to it for now, anyway. One day I'll smoke again, I know I will. I feel like I'm just getting things under control.' Ali paused, 'Hey, and I've got some work as well. They wanted someone to help out at a local shop, selling plants and stuff, bit like the nursery I was at before. It's not much but, well, I need to try and get out a little more and be with people. Desmond's encouraged me to do this. He's given me some details about something called 'Connexions', which helps people, young people, to get into work, or something like that. I know I have to. But it's not going to be easy. It can be difficult coming here.'

'I realise that, Ali, and I know you didn't make it a few times when we first started, but you get here regularly now.'

Ali nodded. 'Yeah. I need to. I know I need to get out more, get used to being out. Spent too long indoors, and in my room. Funny, I don't feel as relaxed as I used to in my room these days. Like I don't want to just lie there like I used to. I need to do something, but if I go out that makes me anxious. It's really difficult.'

'Can't settle at home but anxious if you go out.'

Ali nodded. At least having a couple of beers helped. He'd got into the habit of a few cans of an evening and that seemed to have made a difference. He wasn't planning to mention it, wasn't a problem, just what everyone else did. 'Just got to learn to cope, haven't I?'

'Mhmm, slowly adjust, get used to it.' Ali's attention went back to the diagram on the piece of paper. 'You know, I wish those parts of me weren't so separate. I mean, I wish they weren't in separate bubbles – well, maybe the part of me that gets sad and lonely. I'd like that one to be in such a hard bubble that I can't get into it.' He sighed as he finished speaking.

'So you would like all the others to be less separate but don't want to feel sad and lonely.'

'I hate it.'

Charlotte nodded in response and looked at him, feeling a sudden rush of compassion for him. He had spoken with such pain. 'Sad and lonely, a place you hate to be in.'

'I really do. I don't mind hiding away though sometimes that makes me go into that "sad and lonely" place.'

'I guess the things that make you want to hide away can make you feel sad and lonely as well.'

'Yeah. I'm not always like that. But I can be, and that gets me down. Mum tries to talk to me but I don't want to know. Just want to be left alone. She really tries but I'm not there when I'm like that.'

'Not there?' Charlotte responded with a note of questioning, unsure what Ali meant and inviting him to say a little more.

'No, I just go into myself – the joints used to help – and just float for a while. I can't do that now, I just get heavy and tired now.' He yawned at the thought of it.

'Tired, huh?'

Ali nodded. He had suddenly felt incredibly tired. His eyes felt heavy and his arms felt a little weak. He was aware that his shoulders had tightened again; he tried to loosen them a bit.

'Tight?'

He nodded. He looked at the diagram again. He somehow felt he wanted to draw it differently. 'You know, I don't think that's right. I want to draw it another way.'

'Sure, go ahead. Want another piece of paper?'

Ali nodded and Charlotte reached over for it from the drawer.

'I want more space just for these parts of me.'

Ali described what he was drawing. 'Me in the middle is, was, bullied and hurt. And that can make me want to break free.' He wrote 'Jailbreak'. 'And "Jailbreak" is my way of really getting away. But then, well, I get away when I "hide away" too.' He wrote those words in as well. 'But that makes me depressed, and it makes me sad and lonely.' Ali continued to write, and draw lines connecting up the different feelings. 'But there's a bit of me that's really calm, really, yeah, on top of things.' He wrote 'calm' at the top of the diagram. 'But there's also the anxious me, and that's around all the time.' He wrote 'anxious and panic' to the right. 'But they're not just there, they're kind of everywhere, but not up there where "calm" is.' He wrote them in other places as well. 'Oh yeah, and there's "crazy, paranoid" me as well. Yeah. I get stuck in that.'

Charlotte looked at it. She was struck by how Ali had put boxes round some of the 'parts' or feelings. She invited him to say anything more about what he had drawn and written.

'That's me. No, I need to add voices somewhere. They're in my head but outside as well. I mean, they're me but they sound like they're not me.'

'Mhmm. Where would you want to put them?'

'It's like they come through when I'm here.' He pointed to 'crazy, paranoid'; 'or here,' he was now pointing to 'Jailbreak'. 'And, yeah, I've heard them here as well.' Ali was pointing to 'hide away'.

'So those are the places where you hear voices?'

'I did, but not so much now. But they're all parts of me, aren't they, and all coming from me being bullied.'

'Mhmm. That seems pretty clear, and that's how it has been for you, voices when you hide away, want to break free or feel crazy, paranoid?'

Ali continued to look at what he'd drawn. It seemed strange to be looking at himself. He knew it wasn't himself, not like looking in the mirror or stuff like that, and yet somehow it was like that. He added another word, 'frustration', just above the 'bullied and hurt' part, and then an arrow from 'bullied and hurt' to 'angry', and then to 'crazy, paranoid'. He sat back up again and looked at it. 'Bit of a mess, isn't it?'

'That how it feels?'

Ali nodded. 'But that is me, and I could probably keep adding more, but I want to stop. That's enough. That's what I have to control.' He shook his head. 'All comes from the crap I had in childhood. Bastards!'

'Makes you feel angry?'

Ali looked at the angry part on the drawing. 'Yeah, but look where getting angry takes me?'

'It does if that anger stems from being bullied and hurt.'

'I used to feel hurt, and I guess I still do, but not as much now, well, maybe I still do.' Ali acknowledged to himself that it did still hurt thinking about it, and when he felt he was being bullied now he'd feel hurt and get angry, and frustrated. He looked at the word 'frustration'. Yeah, right along the top of being bullied and hurt. Shit, that was so frustrating when people wouldn't listen to him, wouldn't believe him. He could feel the frustration inside himself as he thought about it. 'I have to change, I have to find a way of getting out of this.'

Charlotte wanted to trust Ali to find his own solutions. She believed that he could, but whether he would, only time would tell. She knew she had to maintain the climate of therapeutic relationship – she sometimes thought of it as 'right relationship' because there was a certain rightness about it, or so it seemed to her. Charlotte noted that Ali's voice had a certain note of desperation to it. At least, that was how she experienced it, although she could not be sure if that was what Ali was experiencing.

'Sounds desperate.'

'How do I get rid of the "bullied and hurt" part of me?'

'That's the bit you want to get rid of?'

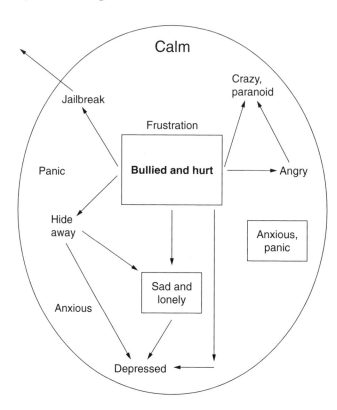

Ali nodded. 'Yeah, if I hadn't been picked on, well, I wouldn't have that part, and maybe all the other parts wouldn't be there. I'd be a different person, you know.'

'Mhmm, a different person to the person that you are.'

'I'd be normal, Charlotte.' He breathed out heavily. 'It makes me feel angry. Just because I was a different colour. Fucking screwed me up, the bastards. Now look at me.' He gestured towards the drawing. 'I want to be normal.' He had raised his voice.

Charlotte nodded her head with a particular intensity. Her voice was deliberately urgent, reflecting the tone of Ali's voice. 'Yeah, you want to be normal.'

'I don't want all of this in my head, it fucks me up.' Ali looked at the drawing again. 'That's what I've got to fight against. I shouldn't have, but I do. And I will. I want that calm.' He smiled as he noted how he had written calm at the top and depressed at the bottom. He hadn't intended it quite like that, but it seemed to sum something up. He knew he had to find that calm. He could, and he did at times, but he usually needed help. The 'hide away' part was a false calm, a delusion. It wasn't really calm. Joints sort of made you feel calm, but he could see that it wasn't really calm, not really, not naturally. He had to stop hiding away, running away, getting depressed, going crazy. He had to find calm, yes, calmness – calmness was the only way out. He shook his head. But he couldn't get out, how could he? He was all of those parts. No, he couldn't get away, but he had to somehow bring them together, be them in a more controlled manner. He would still want to feel angry about things. And, yeah, things would make him sad, and frustrated, and probably depressed. But he wanted to not feel bullied and hurt. That was at the core. He kept coming back to that.

Charlotte had sat with Ali in his silence for a couple of minutes before she responded to what he had last said. 'You want that calm.'

'I want that calm and I want to be free, free like a bird to fly, and not drop into depression, free to fly into the calm air. Yeah, that's what I want. I have to believe that I can fly, I have to.'

'Fly free, fly up into the calm, you have to believe in that.' Charlotte had noticed that the session was coming into the last ten minutes.

'I have to.'

'How about a visualisation to end?'

'Yes, that would be good.'

'Same as before, or something different?' Charlotte was wondering whether a visualisation to help strengthen the sense of flying free might be helpful.

'Don't mind. Up to you.'

'Sure you haven't any preference?'

Ali shook his head. 'I trust you.' And with that he closed his eyes and sat back in the chair.

'OK, so, take a deep breath and in your own time slowly let it out.' Ali did as was being suggested. 'And breathe in again, hold for a moment and out.' Again, Ali breathed in line with the rhythm. 'Imagine that you are a bird, sitting on a nest that has been your home. The sun is shining, the sky is blue, there is a gentle breeze. It ruffles your feathers as you sit and look out over the world.'

Ali sat, it felt good. He could imagine the blue sky vividly after the previous relaxations, and he could imagine the sun on his face.

'You look down and below you is the world, humanity, busily rushing around. People looking stressed, angry, frustrated.' Charlotte paused. Ali could see them, he could imagine the expressions on their faces. He heard Charlotte's voice again. 'Some are sad, some are lonely, some look anxious and try to hide when you look at them.' Ali felt himself smile. This was good. 'Let them go about their business. They do not bother you.' Charlotte paused again, allowing Ali time to engage with the imagery. 'Other people seem to just be going crazy, rushing around, doing crazy things, and still others seem to be just trying to escape, get away from it all. You just look at it all and wonder what is it all about?' Ali felt suddenly quite detached from everything, as though all this was going on but he was somehow not involved, distant somehow, not caught up in it all.

'You turn your gaze upwards, up into the air, up into the blue sky. You feel an urge to fly. You slowly get up and flex your wings. They are long and broad. You stand up on to the edge of the nest and push yourself off, allowing the air to flow under and over your wings. You soar into the cool air, circling, feeling utterly free. You look around you, nothing but sky and air and the sun on your back. And it feels good. You spend a few moments enjoying the freedom of flight.'

Ali could feel himself free. It was a powerful experience. It felt so good.

'Feel the cool, clear air in your lungs as you rhythmically breathe in and out.' Ali felt it. 'Feel yourself turn to the right in the cool air and gradually return to the nest. You soar up to it and at the last moment bring your wings vertical and stop, landing gently.' Another pause. 'Take a few deep breaths and again, in your own time, open your eyes and stretch.'

Ali sat for a few moment's longer. He suddenly took a much deeper breath and slowly opened his eyes. 'That was good. Woo. I was really up there.'

'Good. Take it with you.'

Ali looked at the clock. Time to head off.

'Thanks again. Same time next week?'

'Sure. Just ground yourself a little, you need to be back in touch with the earth.'

Ali pressed his feet into the carpet and stretched again. 'Yeah, that felt good.'

The session ended and Ali headed off, feeling somewhat lightened both physically and in himself. He hoped it would prove to be a good week. He smiled as he thought of all the people in the visualisation, with all his difficulties – angry, crazy people, frustrated. He shook his head. Yes, it felt good.

Counselling session 11: Tuesday 14th July – cannabis dream and a release of anger

Ali did have a good week, although he continued to feel some degree of anxiety most of the time. He was used to it and was learning to get on with his life in spite of it. He had been back to see the psychiatrist in the drug team and they had agreed to reduce his medication. This had started a couple of days ago and so far he was feeling OK. Desmond had been really encouraging. They had explained that they would take it slowly and that he needed to monitor his mood and anything that felt as if he was developing any kind of mental distress.

He had again talked to his mother and felt that his relationship with her had really improved. He also seemed to be spending more time with his brother. They'd drifted apart, but they had spent some time messing around with some computer games and listening to some CDs. It had helped him feel more normal. Just doing normal things, that was what Desmond had said he should concentrate on. So that was what he was trying to do. He had explained this to his mother, and she was very encouraging. But his father still seemed distant and not wanting to really accept that he had changed. He had thawed a little, but it still wasn't an easy relationship.

Ali was sitting opposite Charlotte and looking out of the window. It was raining and had been throughout the day. Ali had got soaked walking from the bus stop. 'Will I ever really get over all the trauma of being picked on and bullied as a child? And is it the reason why I ended up seeing psychiatrists and, well, being in hospital?'

'You want an answer?'

'Seems too simple, really, and, I mean not everyone who's bullied and stuff ends up like this.'

'Mhmm, seems to you that it is too simple.'

For Ali it really did seem that way. And yet he knew he wasn't mad, he could see how he had developed in response to his experiences. And, OK, the cannabis, whilst it had helped in many ways, had seemed to have become more of a problem. 'I mean, I know I'm not mad. Things feel much more under control now. I seem more settled, although I'm not clear yet of feeling anxious about things and it's still not easy to be out sometimes.'

'Mhmm, things are better but not completely resolved, yes?'

'Yes, but will they ever be? I mean, will I really not have this anxiety one day? Will I stop feeling that edginess when I'm in crowded, noisy places, or when I feel like people are looking at me?'

'I honestly can't say, Ali. I believe that people can change and put things behind them, and move on with a different sense of themselves and with different sensitivities, perhaps. But I really do hear and appreciate your wish to know if you will one day lose that edginess in the situations you describe.'

Ali took a deep breath and sighed. 'Sometimes it feels like a constant battle with no real hope of success.'

'And today's one of those days, when it feels like that, constant battle with little hope of success?'

'Rain doesn't help.'

'Gets you down, huh?'

Ali nodded. He'd been feeling better earlier, but as the day had gone on, well, it seemed so grey outside, and he really hadn't felt like coming over for the session. Part of him had wanted to, but another part had wanted him to go back to bed. It hadn't been a voice exactly, not as clear and distinct as he had experienced it in the past, but it did sort of feel like he was being urged not to come. 'Nearly didn't come.'

Charlotte responded by asking him what had been happening for him.

'Dunno, just felt like I couldn't be bothered.'

'Couldn't be bothered to come over, yeah?'

Ali had mixed feelings. He liked Charlotte. In a way he didn't want to let her down, but he also wanted to do what he wanted to do. He'd wanted to stay in bed. 'Wanted to stay in bed.'

'Mhmm, you just felt like you'd rather stay in bed.' Charlotte waited to see in what direction Ali wanted to take the session.

'Just couldn't be bothered. Just wanted to be under the duvet.'

'Mhmm, under the duvet and not bother.'

Ali yawned. 'Just wanted to hide away, that's all I can say, I think that the "hide away" part of me wanted that to happen.'

'Mhmm, the "hide away" part of you didn't want you here but you're here so that part didn't really get control.'

'No, it didn't. I didn't let it. I pulled myself together and got out of the house. It wasn't easy. I mean, it really wasn't easy.'

Charlotte wondered what had made the difference, what had enabled Ali to get up and out of the house and make his way over to the session. However, she noted the urge to question but let it go, allowing Ali to continue to decide the content and focus of the session.

'It wasn't easy, you really had to, what, make yourself come?'

'Sort of. Mum reminded me this morning before she went off to work. She's still very encouraging. And I said yes, and I felt good, felt sure I'd come over. Didn't experience any reason why not.'

'So, all OK this morning then.'

'Well, not sure about all OK. Had a bad night last night. Kind of disturbing. Didn't think too much of it this morning but kept thinking about it later.'

'So something disturbed you and you ended up thinking about it.'

'Yeah. It'll probably sound crazy, but, well, I don't know where I was or what I was doing, but I was with a lot of people. Not sure if I knew them. Anyway, there was some pot being handed around and, well, I had some. Funny, though, I tried not to in the dream but in the end smoked a couple of joints. It felt so vivid, I mean, really vivid, like I was smoking for real. It was a wonderful dream but I woke up this morning feeling like I used to when I was smoking, you know? I mean, I really was. Same kind of sensations in my head, but I knew I hadn't had anything.'

'So you knew you hadn't smoked a joint or two.'

'That's right, but then, well, I felt sure that I had, I mean really convinced. I could smell it, taste it, feel the sensations in my head, I mean, well, if I'd been anywhere else with any friends who smoked then I'd know I'd have tried it. But I didn't, I really didn't, but I felt like I had.'

'You knew you hadn't but you sure felt like you had.' Charlotte recognised the features of a typical substance use dream. She'd heard drinkers talk of 'drinking dreams' (Bryant-Jefferies, 2001, 2003a) and this sounded similar, but simply related to the experience of smoking cannabis. She knew how vivid they could be, and how unsettling, leaving people with genuinely experienced symptoms and effects of having used the substance in their dream experience.

'Really got to me. Mum thought I'd been back on the pot again. Said I looked really out of it. That's how I felt, but I hadn't.'

Charlotte explained about these kinds of dream and sought to reassure Ali that they could happen and could seem very real. But that it was important to try and not act on them.

'Does my head in all of this. I mean, what's that all about?'

'Drugs generate intense experiences. Seems that the brain, through our dreams, can cause us to relive the experience.'

'Really left me craving a joint.'

'Mhmm, left you craving, like you were back in touch with that experience.'

Ali nodded. It had been really unsettling. 'Something else I've got to get over?'

Charlotte nodded. 'Yes.'

Ali was tight-lipped as he thought about it. 'All this stuff in my head.' He felt angry and frustrated. He wanted to move on, get a grip on his life. He knew things had to be different. He was making changes, but it was so difficult. He could feel so anxious and panicky. 'If only I could take something to settle me down.'

'Mhmm, something to make you feel more settled.'

'But Desmond says no. Says I need to adjust, that it takes time, but that I will settle down.' He shook his head and breathed deeply. 'I wouldn't want much. Just take the edge off things.'

'Mhmm, so the idea of taking something to calm you down you feel would help?'

'Yeah, I do.' Ali paused. 'But then, well, then I'd be relying on something again and Desmond says be at risk of developing another addiction. And he doesn't want that to happen.'

'So, he doesn't want you to take that risk of developing another addiction.' Charlotte did not want to take sides on this, but to continue to simply empathise with Ali and his feelings and thoughts around this issue. She well appreciated where Desmond was coming from, and she also felt for Ali as well. It was a difficult one, but she knew the importance of learning how to cope without the chemical crutch, as it were. She also recognised that for some people the need was such that they did require ongoing medication. However, Ali was being reduced on his medication at the moment, to try and enable him to in a sense experience himself for real. It then became a question of whether he could hold himself together in the face of the reality of his own experience.

'No, he doesn't. And, well, just a little, I mean, I'm not asking much. Can you talk to him? I don't seem to be able to get through to him.'

Charlotte knew that this wasn't her role. She recognised the desperation in Ali's voice.

How does the person-centred counsellor respond to a client's direct request for them to in a sense act as an advocate on their behalf? What impact would it have on their relationship if Charlotte was to agree to this, or if she did not? It is a sensitive time. People can feel quite powerless sometimes, feeling that other people involved in their care or treatment are not listening to them. But what should the counsellor do?

'I really do hear you saying you want medication to help calm you down. And I know you are already reducing what you have been taking. Can't be easy.'

'Bloody hard. I really wish it was easier.'

'Mhmm, and that wish for it to be easier sounds very present at the moment.'

'I just want to stop feeling like this. I found a way to deal with it, but I'm told I can't do that. And now the medication – which did help a bit – well, now I have to reduce that. And it just feels too much.'

'Too much to reduce the medication you're on when you can't use the pot any more.'

'Well, I mean, I could, but, well, I know I can't, but I want to, I really want to.'

'That urge is so strong in you at the moment.'

'I just want to feel better', Ali was staring down at the carpet. He felt miserable. He just seemed to swing so much inside himself at the moment, but now it all just seemed too much. What was the point? Why bother? To hell with everyone, he wanted a joint, he wanted to get some relief.

Charlotte nodded, 'Yeah, to feel better.'

At least Charlotte seemed to be listening to him, wasn't telling him what was good for him. He'd had enough of that, got that from his father all the time. He felt quite pissed off with Desmond at times. At other times, he really understood where he was coming from, but just at this moment he was feeling pissed off. 'Desmond really does piss me off.'

Charlotte nodded, 'Pisses you off'. She kept her response simple and waited to see if Ali was going to express these feelings, or just talk about them. She sensed that perhaps things had built up and maybe Ali needed to connect with his feelings, make them visible, have them heard and accepted.

'Well, yeah, I mean, shit, I can't take it, you know, it really gets to me.'

'Mhmm, not sure you can take it.'

'I mean, I don't want to go back to hospital again. Shit, that was horrible. I'm not mad. I just want to feel normal. Why can't I feel normal? I just want something to help me.' He felt desperate, felt feelings emerging as he spoke. It felt like a nightmare that he couldn't escape from. He needed something, anything, to feel better.

'You need something to take away the discomfort, you mean?'

'Yeah...' He paused. 'Well, yeah, I do, but I'm not going to get it, am I?'

Charlotte shook her head. 'It's a tough time, Ali, and, well, maybe you need more support, more contact with people to support and encourage you at the moment?'

'I need something. Yeah, I guess I do want to run and hide, get away from it all.' He looked over at the diagram that Charlotte had put out again on the table. 'It's me just wanting to hide away, all the time, that seems what I want to do. And I can't, not if I want to change. But it's so hard, Charlotte, so hard.'

'Hard to change, hard to not let that "hide away" part of you take over.' She had noticed Ali look over at the diagram.

'I feel it so much. It's like instinctive. Run away, get away, hide away, don't face up to it. But I have to.' Ali's thoughts slipped back into his own past. He hadn't been able to face up to the bullies at school, not for a long while. He breathed deeply and sighed as he thought back to those times. He felt a surge of anger and felt his jaw tightening. 'I really hate those bastards for screwing me up. Mum says I should forgive them. Says it is what Allah would want me to do.' He shook his head. 'I can't and I don't want to. I wish I could beat the shit out of them. Bastards, all of them.' He clenched his fists as he spoke.

'You'd really like to beat the shit out of the bastards.' Charlotte spoke slowly, empathising with what Ali had said and was feeling.

'They've made my life a fucking misery and fucked me up.' He shook his head again. He snorted. Yeah, he did want to beat the shit out of them, but, well, he also knew they had just been kids. But he still wanted to smash them. The constant verbal he got from them, being picked on, pushed around, having pranks played on him that weren't jokes and weren't funny. He took a deep breath as he thought back. He could see their faces, clearly, and hear their words. They still hurt, he still hurt. He couldn't forgive them. They fucked him up, they were responsible. And yet, as he sat there shaking his head, he also knew as well that somehow he had to let go of them, of it all. He had to move on. He had to somehow stop being so sensitive, but he couldn't help it. It was how he was. Another deep breath and a sigh. The thought of being like this the rest of his life. No, he couldn't cope with that. He had to be different, he had to. He couldn't go on like this. It was all too damn painful. He closed his eyes as he felt the mix of anger and desperation in his head and in his body. He was feeling tense, he was still clenching his fists. Another deep breath. He felt sure he'd feel better if he could get his anger and frustration out of his system.

'Oh fuck it, fuck it, fuck it. I've had enough of those bastards.' He sighed loudly. 'I want them out of my head, I want it all out of my head.' He slammed his right fist down on the chair arm. He knew he wanted to smash something, and he knew that it was a familiar reaction to the frustration he often felt. He slammed his fist down again, and kept doing it, thump, thump, thump, thump. He continued to pound away, his jaw set firm. He lifted his hand and held it, suspended above the chair arm, his fist so tight, his fingernails digging into the palm of his hand. There were a couple of cushions in the corner of the room. Charlotte wondered about suggesting he hit them, but there was something about that rhythmic thump, the sound, maybe that was important and she didn't want to disrupt or disturb what Ali was needing to do.

'Yeah, get them out of your head.'

Ali was taking a deep breath as he continued to hold his clenched fist above the chair arm. He didn't really hear Charlotte, at least he heard her voice but he wasn't listening. He thought of the kids at school, their fucking white faces jeering at him. He'd wipe that jeer off their faces, how he'd wanted to do that but hadn't been able to. Why had they lived in a place that was so fucking white? His father, he'd had to move there because of his job. Bastard. He was to blame. He was to fucking blame. He smashed his fist down again, now his feelings had become more frustration than anger. He leant back in the chair. Nobody had been there for him, he'd had to deal with it on his own. It was his father's fault, he was to blame. He was to blame.

He opened his eyes and continued to clench his teeth together. 'He didn't think about me, just his precious, fucking job.' Another deep sigh.

Charlotte guessed Ali was talking about his father, although she knew this was an assumption. But she wasn't going to check this out, she needed to empathise and accept what Ali was thinking and feeling. 'That's how it feels, only his precious, fucking job mattered.'

Ali shook his head. Another deep breath and he felt himself relax as he breathed out, blowing the air forcefully through his nose. He dropped his shoulders, he couldn't hold the tension in his body any more. Maybe he couldn't hold his feelings any more. He shook his head as he sighed again. It felt as though the anger had eased a little, at least momentarily. 'Guess he had to do it . . .' Ali was shaking his head though, still not really wanting to accept it. 'I just wish someone had been there for me.'

For Charlotte it seemed as though the atmosphere suddenly changed. From an electric tension suddenly it seemed as though Ali had suddenly become like a small boy. 'Yes, if only someone had been there for you.' She realised she had tightened her own lips. She nodded and took a deep breath herself. 'If only . . .' The last two words were not an empathic response, but an expression of her own reaction.

Ali blew a sharp breath out of his nose and shook his head himself. 'If only things had been different.' He felt strangely calm, kind of numb as he sat still shaking his head, thinking about his past in a general and non-specific kind of way.

Charlotte nodded. She didn't say anything. She had already empathised. She allowed Ali the space and time to simply be with what he was now experiencing. She didn't want to say anything that might distract him from the focus that had emerged for him, that might take him out of the thoughts and feelings that had become present for him.

Ali swallowed. He felt sad, very sad as he thought of the crap he'd had to put up with. There were tears in his eyes. He took a deep breath and breathed out with a sigh. He felt suddenly quite weak. There was a kind of calmness as well but he wasn't really thinking about that. He just sat, breathing deeply every now and then and still shaking his head, his right hand now across his face, his elbow supported by his left hand.

Ali dropped his hand over his mouth and looked up, opening his eyes and looking across at Charlotte. 'He had to do it, he didn't have a choice.' Another deep breath and a sigh. 'He had to go with his job, it was just . . .' He shook his head. He didn't know how to put into words what he was feeling. He shook his head again.

'It was just . . . ?' Charlotte empathised and by so doing and with her tone of voice, invited Ali to say more, if he could.

'I don't know how to say it. Just wish he could have been a bit more sensitive. But he wasn't. It was just a bad time and, well, I had to get on with it.' He stretched in the chair, he was very stiff, and immediately yawned. He felt tired. Tired of it all. Tired of how he was. Just tired. He shook his head again. 'I feel better for all of this, somehow. Feel like I've burnt something out of myself.' Another deep breath, and a yawn. 'Feels like it's been a long time.'

Charlotte wasn't sure whether Ali was talking about his life or the session. But she decided it was not important to clarify this, she simply empathised with the sense of 'long time' that he had mentioned. 'Mhmm, seems like a long time.' Seems like a long time. Words of a song came to her. She let a line or two pass through her head, 'seems like a long time, seems like a long time, seems like a long, long time.' She pushed the words aside.

Another deep breath from Ali, deeper than previously. 'Yeah.' He swallowed. 'Yeah.'

They sat, the silence remained between them. Ali feeling suddenly very quiet and still, and reflective, although he wasn't really thinking, at least he was, but the thoughts were sort of passing through his mind without him really engaging with them.

For Charlotte, the words of the song had come back.

Good times are only, the other side of bad times, and if you've ever wished bad times would pass.
You know what it's like, to wish good times would come and don't it
Seem like a long time. Seem like a long time. Seem like a long, long time.
And don't it, seem like a long time, seem like a long time, seem like a long, long time.

Night times are only, the other side of day times, and if you've ever waited for dawn to come . . .*

Charlotte pulled herself out of the song in her head. She'd drifted away from Ali. She glanced at the clock, it was nearly time for the session to end. She looked across at him. He looked as though he had worn himself out.

'You look tired, maybe seems like a long time, it's been a heavy session.'

Ali nodded. 'Yeah, but I feel better for it.' A deep breath. 'Yeah, I think I needed it. I feel calmer somehow. Don't suppose it'll last, but I do feel calmer just now.' He paused as he realised it was a bit like how he had felt after the relaxations. 'You know, it's weird, but it's a bit like how I feel after the relaxations we've done.'

Charlotte felt herself smiling in response. 'Well, you wanted to find that calmness in yourself, maybe today you have found another way.'

---

* 'Seems Like a Long Time', written by T Anderson from the album *Every Picture Tells a Story*, by Rod Stewart.

Ali nodded. He was suddenly aware of feeling very hungry, his stomach was gnawing at him. He needed to eat.

'Guess I'd better head off.'

'Sure. Look after yourself, Ali, you'll be feeling more sensitive just at the moment. Big noisy world out there. Maybe take a while to just prepare yourself to head out.' Charlotte felt it important to remind clients of this, particularly after this kind of session. People could go out still in a sensitive state and be powerfully affected by the noise and bustle out in the street. It could disorientate them.

'Sure. Thanks. I'll take my time. Feel like I need to go somewhere and just think for a bit.'

'I'm sure you'll know what you need to do.'

Ali nodded. Yes, he knew he needed to be quiet. He'd go for a walk, get away from the High Street. He left and Charlotte sat down to reflect on the session. It had been a tough one. Lots of feelings, lots of intensity. Ali had clearly burned up a lot of energy. He'd connected with feelings about his past, the kids who'd picked on him, his father. He hadn't said anything about his mother or brother who, of course, had also contributed to his not feeling he was given the time and attention he needed. But maybe the feelings associated with that would come out another time.

She didn't know just how he was going to react to the session. He certainly looked as though he had a lot to think about. She trusted that this was timely. She accepted that she never knew from session to session what would happen and she wasn't an expert in knowing ahead of time what was best for her clients. Her role was to create a therapeutic space and offer a quality of relationship that could facilitate her client's inner process. She accepted wholeheartedly that Rogers was right, that there was an actualising tendency within all of us, that sought to maximise the individual's capacity for satisfying experiences. She knew this had different meanings and emphasis for different people, that it depended largely on where their consciousness was focused. Everyone was different but everyone essentially wanted to feel 'good', or feel 'better', though that meant different things to different people. For one person it could mean looking at a sunset, for someone else it could mean finding relief by cutting themselves. She shook her head as she thought of the contrast between these two extremes. People did what they needed to do to feel what they needed to feel. And therein lies the human story and, for so many, the human tragedy as well.

She thought of the notion of an actualising tendency. It wasn't a good or a bad tendency, it just was, a something that urged development. It could take people in so many different directions. For some, the satisfaction of a complex life, for others the satisfaction of greater simplicity. But it kept people moving, and yet it could keep people stuck as well, hold them in a place in themselves or in their lives that they did not want to move away from. A force that perhaps our own individual states of mind and heart gave direction to, if force was the right word for it. No, it wasn't a force acting on something, it was an essential ingredient of creation. She thought of the Tao, the notion of flow, of going with some unseen flow. The Flow of Life? She wasn't sure exactly what she meant.

She took a deep breath as her thoughts turned to those who through traumatic experience, or as a result of chemical imbalances within their brains, were driven to derive satisfaction from actions that caused themselves, or others, pain and hurt. If pain was all you ever knew, and if psychologically that had been symbolised as normal to the point that pain and hurt were linked to that individual's primary sense of self, then they may well act in ways in order to maintain that sense of self. What did that mean? How would the actualising tendency work with that?

Her thoughts went back to Ali. How would things shape up for him? She felt he had made a lot of progress, that he really was opening up to himself, and learning – albeit painfully – to cope without recourse to the cannabis. But she appreciated it wasn't easy. And there was still uncertainty as to his mental health, how he would be as the medication he was taking was reduced. Was his symptomology simply a result of his early-life experiences, or was there a chemical process that also needed a chemical intervention to help him maintain long-term stability? That was assuming that stability was a good thing anyway. She thought of all the artists, composers, poets and others, of course, whose creativity was intimately linked to their instability. She wondered how many significant figures from the past might have been less significant had they been given medication to cope with mood swings.

She hoped Ali would continue to work at coming to terms with his past and with his shift of mood and inner experiencing. She looked at the diagram on the table – a kind of mind/emotion map. She knew it was incomplete. The complexity of the human psyche could not easily be fitted on to a sheet of A4 paper. The subtle connections, the many different parts that made up the whole that was an individual and unique person. She took out the file and wrote her notes for the session.

Summary

Ali wants something to help him feel better, to quell the discomfort he feels. He connects with feelings towards his past, towards the children who picked on him, and towards his father. He releases anger and frustration in the session and comes around in himself towards a clearer realisation that his father had to move the family because of work, which meant Ali went to the school where he was so bullied and taunted for his colour. He is left feeling calmer. He leaves the session needing to have quiet space in which to reflect on his experience.

Points for discussion

- Evaluate Charlotte's responses to Ali. How do you view her style?
- Where might you have responded differently, and why?
- What has struck you as being the key moments in Ali's therapeutic process?

- How much communication is necessary between a counsellor and a key-worker in a multi-disciplinary setting and in a situation typified by a client such as Ali?
- What do you feel to be the next therapeutic steps for Ali to take?
- If you were Charlotte, what would you be taking to supervision, and why?
- How should a counsellor respond when a client requests them to take on an advocacy role? On what basis would you accept or decline this request?
- Write your own notes for the session.

Author's epilogue

Perhaps, by the time Ali has reached his next session his mother, Fareeda, will have ended her counselling, or perhaps for her it is just the beginning of a longer process as she finds other aspects of herself that she wants to explore, understand and perhaps redefine. She is beginning to see the son she once knew, although whether he evidences this as he grows into adulthood, only time will tell. For Ali, the counselling process may continue for some time yet, but he is now facing his next challenge, of reducing the medication. Will therapy be enough to enable him to resolve the fragmentation within his structure of self? Will the voices fade, and the paranoia lose its strength? Will he be able to become truly centred in a more integrated sense of his own personhood? What new feature of his personality might emerge over time and through new experiences in the future?

How will mother and son relate to each other as they go through the changes that are likely to occur as a result of their counselling? It is tempting to wonder just how much they will recognise in each other by the time they have each completed their respective therapeutic processes.

This book, as they all have in the Living Therapy series, took its own direction. I set out with an idea, that of a mother going to counselling to seek support in relation to her struggle to cope with a son with symptoms that could be attributable to mental illness and whose use of cannabis seemed to be increasingly problematic. Issues of race and religious difference emerged within the sessions with Fareeda, and the strength and importance of her faith became revealed. Carla, the counsellor, learned from this experience, opening her heart and mind to Fareeda's view of life, including her need to be reassured that she was serving the will of Allah.

As is so often the case, things got worse for her son before they started to get better. Ali had a psychotic episode, was taken into hospital, stabilised and then began the long and arduous process of trying to maintain some degree of abstinence from the cannabis, whilst also gaining deeper insight into himself. It took him a while to attend counselling consistently, he lived out some of the inner dramas locked within the parts that together formed his structure of self. Charlotte, his counsellor, was stretched at times as she sought to stay with Ali as he moved in and out of a frame of reference that was simply beyond the horizon of her own experience.

Both counsellors utilised their respective supervisors, making sense of what they were experiencing with their clients, seeking to resolve issues that arose for them and preparing themselves to continue with the therapeutic work.

I hope that this book has contained and conveyed some ideas around how the person-centred approach to counselling and psychotherapy can be applied to working with people who are experiencing 'psychotic' symptomology. Like others, I am convinced that psychotic symptoms may well be chaotic attempts by a person who is in a state of psychological fragmentation to try and achieve some degree of self-healing. Psychosis is surely the parts being made visible – distressing perhaps to the client, though often more so to those close to them. The instinctive reaction is to contain and manage, to try and remove the symptoms. But perhaps that is the opposite to what is needed. Perhaps the inner experiencing needs to be allowed to exist in awareness with the client being offered warm acceptance and empathic sensitivity to what is becoming present.

If the human person is subject to an actualising tendency, as Rogers suggests, and if this inner urge is constantly seeking to bring the person towards a more fulfilling and satisfying set of experiences, involving greater personal integration, then surely the true healing process must involve creating the relational environment in which this tendency can most productively operate in bringing about constructive personality change. Mental illness covers a broad spectrum of experiencing. There will be those for whom the root cause is a chemical or organic problem requiring a chemical or organic solution. However, whilst symptomologies may be similar, causes may differ. The challenge for mental health professionals, including counsellors and psychotherapists, lies in recognising in what area of the person, or the person's experience, the cause of the problem arises and therefore what type of response, or set of responses, is likely to be most helpful. It seems to me that the person-centred approach, stressing the hugely important relational element in the healing process, must play a significant part in effective responding to human experiencing that exists under the category of 'mental illness'.

I will end with a quote from Peggy Natiello, who writes in her book *The Person-Centred Approach: a passionate presence* of her mother's experience of developing severe psychotic symptoms. She describes her psychiatrist as being 'competent, ingratiating and, in the interest of maintaining clear professional boundaries, personally distant'. She writes of how near the beginning of a therapy session the psychiatrist began sobbing uncontrollably. He disclosed to her mother how one of his children had committed suicide. She writes: 'I was not there, but I am sure that my profoundly empathic mother became the *healer* during the remainder of that session. More importantly, Dr Sands brought his genuine, vulnerable self into the relationship, probably because he could not repress it. His presence as a real person, the balance of power between him and my mother, and, consequently, their personal connection changed markedly. From that time forward, their work *together* became more effective and healing. I suspected then, and have since become convinced in my practice of psychotherapy, that an authentic, connected relationship between client and therapist has considerable impact on healing and therapeutic outcome' (Natiello, 2001, p. 26).

References

Ali A (1938) *The Meaning of the Glorious Qur'ān* (3e). Dar Al-Kitab Al-Masri, Cairo.

Asay T and Lambert M (1999) The empirical case for common factors in therapy. In: M Hubble, B Duncan and S Miller (eds) *The Heart and Soul of Therapy*. American Psychological Association Press, Washington, DC.

Bentall R (1990) The syndromes and symptoms of psychosis. In: R Bentall (ed.) *Reconstructing Schizophrenia*. Routledge, London.

Bozarth J (1998) *Person-Centred Therapy: a revolutionary paradigm*. PCCS Books, Ross-on-Wye.

Bozarth J (2002) Empirically supported treatments: epitomy of the specificity myth. In: J Watson, R Goldman and M Warner (eds) *Client-centred and Experiential Psychotherapy in the 21st century: advances in theory, research and practice*. PCCS Books, Ross-on-Wye, pp. 168–81.

Bozarth J and Wilkins P (eds) (2001) *Rogers' Therapeutic Conditions: evolution, theory and practice*. Volume 3: *Congruence*. PCCS Books, Ross-on-Wye.

Bryant-Jefferies R (2001) *Counselling the Person Beyond the Alcohol Problem*. Jessica Kingsley Publishers, London.

Bryant-Jefferies R (2003a) *Counselling a Recovering Drug User: a person-centred dialogue*. Radcliffe Medical Press, Oxford.

Bryant-Jefferies R (2003b) *Counselling Young People: person-centred dialogues*. Radcliffe Medical Press, Oxford.

Bryant-Jefferies R (2003c) *Time-Limited Therapy in Primary Care: a person-centred dialogue*. Radcliffe Medical Press, Oxford.

Bryant-Jefferies R (2004) *Counselling for Progressive Disability: person-centred dialogues*. Radcliffe Medical Press, Oxford.

Curtis Jenkins G (2002) Good money after bad? The justification for the expansion of counselling services in primary health care. In: C Feltham (ed.) *What's the Good of Counselling & Psychotherapy?* Sage, London.

Deleu C and Van Werde D (1998) The relevance of a phenomenological attitude when working with psychotic people. In: B Thorne and E Lambers (eds) *Person-Centred Therapy: a European perspective*. Sage, London, pp. 206–16.

Embleton Tudor L, Keemar K, Tudor K *et al.* (2004) *The Person-Centred Approach: a contemporary introduction*. Palgrave MacMillan, Basingstoke.

Evans R (1975) *Carl Rogers: the man and his ideas*. Dutton and Co., New York.

Gaylin N (2001) *Family, Self and Psychotherapy: a person-centred perspective*. PCCS Books, Ross-on-Wye.

Hallam R (1983) Agoraphobia: deconstructing a clinical syndrome. *Bulletin of British Psychological Society*. 36: 337–40.

Hallam R (1989) Classification and research into panic. In: R Baker and M McFadyen (eds) *Panic Disorder*. Wiley, Chichester.

Hallett R (1990) Melancholia and depression. A brief history and analysis of contemporary confusions. Unpublished Masters thesis, University of East London.

Haugh S and Merry T (eds) (2001) *Rogers' Therapeutic Conditions: evolution, theory and practice. Volume 2: Empathy*. PCCS Books, Ross-on-Wye.

Karon B and Vanderbos G (1981) *Psychotherapy of Schizophrenia*. Aaronson, New York.

Kutchins H and Kirk S (1997) *Making us Crazy: DSM: the psychiatric bible and the creation of mental disorders*. The Free Press/Simon Schuster, New York.

Lambers E (1994) Personality disorder. In: D Mearns (ed.) *Developing Person-Centred Counselling*. Sage, London.

Lambers E (1994) Psychosis. In: D Mearns (ed.) *Developing Person-Centred Counselling*. Sage, London.

Mearns D (1990) The counsellor's experience of success. In: D Mearns and W Dryden (eds) *Experiences of Counselling in Action*. Sage, London.

Mearns D (1999) Person-centred therapy with configurations of self. *Counselling*. 10: 125–30.

Mearns D (2000) The nature of 'configurations' within self. In: D Mearns and B Thorne (eds) *Person-Centred Therapy Today*. Sage, London.

Mearns D and Thorne B (1988) *Person-Centred Counselling in Action*. Sage, London.

Mearns D and Thorne B (1999) *Person-Centred Counselling in Action (2e)*. Sage, London.

Mearns D and Thorne B (2000) *Person-Centred Therapy Today*. Sage, London.

Merry T (2002) *Learning and Being in Person-Centred Counselling (2e)*. PCCS Books, Ross-on-Wye.

Miller W and Rollnick S (1991) *Motivational Interviewing: preparing people to change addictive behaviour*. Guilford Press, New York.

Natiello P (2001) *The Person-Centred Approach: a passionate presence*. PCCS Books, Ross-on-Wye.

National Treatment Agency (2002) *Models of Care for Treatment of Adult Drug Misusers*. National Treatment Agency, London.

Patterson CH (2000) *Understanding Psychotherapy: fifty years of client-centred theory and practice*. PCCS Books, Ross-on-Wye.

Pörtner M (2000) *Trust and Understanding: the person-centred approach to everyday care for people with special needs*. PCCS Books, Ross-on-Wye.

Prouty G (2002) The practice of pre-therapy. In: G Wyatt and P Sanders (eds) *Rogers' Therapeutic Conditions: evolution, theory and practice. Volume 4: Contact and perception*. PCCS Books, Ross-on-Wye.

Prouty G, Van Werde D and Pörtner M (2002) *Pre-Therapy: reaching contact-impaired clients.* PCCS Books, Ross-on-Wye.

Rogers C (1946) Significant aspects of client-centred therapy. *American Psychologist.* 1: 415–22.

Rogers C (1951) *Client-Centred Therapy.* Constable, London.

Rogers C (1957) The necessary and sufficient conditions of therapeutic personality change. *Journal of Consulting Psychology.* 21: 95–103.

Rogers C (1959) A theory of therapy, personality and interpersonal relationships as developed in the client-centred framework. In: S Koch (ed.) *Psychology: a study of a science.* Volume 3: *Formulations of the person and the social context.* McGraw-Hill, New York, pp. 185–246.

Rogers C (1961) *On Becoming a Person: a therapist's view of psychotherapy.* Constable and Co., London.

Rogers C (1970) *On Encounter Groups.* Harper and Row, New York.

Rogers C (1980) *A Way of Being.* Houghton-Mifflin, Boston, MA.

Rogers C (1986) A client-centered/person-centered approach to therapy. In: I Kutash and A Wolfe (eds) *Psychotherapists' Casebook.* Jossey Bass, San Francisco, pp. 236–57.

Rogers C (1986) The Rust Workshop: a personal overview. *Journal of Humanistic Psychology.* 26(3): 23–45.

Rogers C (1987) Inside the world of the Soviet professional. *Journal of Humanistic Psychology.* 27(3).

Rogers C and Stevens B (1973) *Person to Person: the problem of being human.* Souvenir Press, London. Originally published in 1967 by Real People Press, USA.

Rogers C, Gendlin E, Kiesler D *et al.* (eds) (1967) *The Therapeutic Relationship and its Impact. A study of psychotherapy with schizophrenics.* University of Wisconsin Press, Wisconsin.

Schlien J (1961) A client-centred approach to schizophrenia: first approximation. In: C Rogers and B Stevens (eds) *Person to Person: the problem of being human.* Souvenir Press, London, pp. 151–65.

Slade P and Cooper R (1979) Some difficulties with the term 'schizophrenia': an alternative model. *British Journal of Social and Clinical Psychology.* 18: 309–17.

Sommerbeck L (2003) *The Client-Centred Therapist in Psychiatric Contexts: a therapist's guide to the psychiatric landscape and its inhabitants.* PCCS Books, Ross-on-Wye.

Tudor K and Worrall M (2004) *Freedom to Practise: person-centred approaches to supervision.* PCCS Books, Ross-on-Wye.

Van Werde D (1998) Anchorage as a core concept in working with psychotic people. In: B Thorne and E Lambers (eds) *Person-Centred Therapy: a European perspective.* Sage, London, pp. 195–205.

Vincent S (2005) *Being Empathic: a companion for counsellors and therapists.* Radcliffe Publishing, Oxford.

Warner M (2000) Person-centred therapy at the difficult edge: a developmentally based model of fragile and dissociated process. In: D Mearns and B Thorne (eds) *Person-Centred Therapy Today.* Sage, London.

Warner M (2002) Psychological contact, meaningful process and human nature. In: G Wyatt and P Sanders (eds) *Rogers' Therapeutic Conditions: evolution, theory and practice*. Volume 4: *Contact and perception*. PCCS Books, Ross-on-Wye, pp. 76–95.

Wiener M (1989) Psychopathology reconsidered. Depression interpreted as psychosocial interactions. *Clinical Psychology Review*. 9: 295–321.

Wilkins P (2003) *Person Centred Therapy in Focus*. Sage, London.

Wyatt G (ed.) (2001) *Rogers' Therapeutic Conditions: evolution, theory and practice*. Volume 1: *Congruence*. PCCS Books, Ross-on-Wye.

Wyatt G and Sanders P (eds) (2002) *Rogers' Therapeutic Conditions: evolution, theory and practice*. Volume 4: *Contact and perception*. PCCS Books, Ross-on-Wye.

Index